Low-Carb Smoothies

ALSO BY DONNA PLINER RODNITZKY

Ultimate Smoothies

Summer Smoothies

Slim Smoothies

Tipsy Smoothies

The Ultimate Low-Carb
Diet Cookbook

Ultimate Juicing

Sinful Smoothies

Low-Carb Smoothies

More Than 135 Recipes
to Satisfy Your Sweet Tooth
Without Guilt

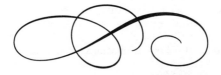

Donna Pliner
Rodnitzky

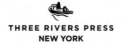

THREE RIVERS PRESS
NEW YORK

Various recipes have been previously published
in slightly different form in the following works
by the author: *Ultimate Juicing* (Prima, 2000),
Ultimate Smoothies (Prima, 2000), *Summer
Smoothies* (Prima, 2002), *Slim Smoothies*
(Prima, 2003), *Tipsy Smoothies* (Three Rivers
Press, 2003), and *Sinful Smoothies* (Three
Rivers Press, 2004)

Library of Congress Cataloging-in-Publication
Data

Rodnitzky, Donna.
   Low-carb smoothies : more than 135 recipes
to satisfy your sweet tooth without guilt / Donna
Pliner Rodnitzky. — 1st ed.
   1. Blenders (Cookery) 2. Smoothies (Beverages)
I. Title.
   TX840.B5R62694   2005
   641.8'75—dc22   2004021277

ISBN 1-4000-8230-7

Printed in the United States of America

Design by Karen Minster

10 9 8 7 6 5 4 3 2 1

FIRST EDITION

*It's impossible
to express in words*

the appreciation and admiration

I have for my husband, Bob.

He has been my rock

for more than thirty-five years.

It is because of his encouragement and

continuous belief in all my endeavors

that I have been able to write

Low-Carb Smoothies

as well as my other cookbooks.

My wonderful children,

David, Adam, and Laura,

continue to astound me with their

wit, character, adventuresome spirit,

and pursuit of excellence.

They are an inspiration

for me always to aim higher.

Acknowledgments

I WOULD LIKE TO THANK my editor, Caroline Sincerbeaux, who has been a joy to work with this past year. I have been impressed with her relentless enthusiasm, insightful suggestions, and extraordinary eye for detail. My gratitude also goes to Karen Minster for designing such a beautiful book, and to the entire staff at Three Rivers Press for their excellent professionalism in bringing this book to publication.

Contents

Introduction

*A diet is the penalty we pay
for exceeding the feed limit.*

— ANONYMOUS

IN THE 1970S, DR. ROBERT C. ATKINS PUBLISHED the book *Dr. Atkins' Diet Revolution*. This book revolutionized the way millions of people dieted. Instead of encouraging us to restrict the amount of fat in our diet as most diet experts stressed at that time, Dr. Atkins told us to focus on reducing the daily intake of refined carbohydrates. He was convinced that dietary carbohydrates were the main culprit in causing people to gain weight, largely because carbohydrate-laden foods such as sugars and starches cause the body to increase the production of insulin, a hormone that promotes fat accumulation in the body.

While most people credit Dr. Atkins for introducing the low-carb diet, this way of eating can actually be traced back to England in the 1860s. It began with the dietary dilemma of an undertaker named William Banting, who was 5 feet 5 inches tall and weighed 202 pounds. Because of this excessive weight he couldn't bend over, and any exertion left him exhausted. Since obesity was rare at that time, he was subject to public ridicule. His doctors suggested diuretics and Turkish baths, but by the time he was sixty-six years old, he had resigned himself to the belief that he would be obese until the day he died.

His fate changed when his physician returned from a seminar on diabetes that suggested a high-protein, low-carbohydrate diet, usually recommended for diabetics, might also have an effect on obesity. Mr. Banting was told to eliminate bread, potatoes, beer, milk, sugar, and butter from his daily meal plan. While he continued to eat his customary four meals a day, he followed the diet and successfully lost forty-six pounds in less than a year. Banting was so elated with his success that he wanted to share it with the public. He wrote and distributed a twenty-two-page pamphlet entitled "Letter on Corpulence" that warned against eating foods that contained sugar and starch. Because of the immediate and overwhelmingly positive response to the first thousand copies of his publication, he printed and sold another fifty thousand. Not surprisingly, the medical community immediately attacked the diet and criticized it for not being studied to their satisfaction (sound familiar?). Mr. Banting, for his part, went on to live to be eighty-one years old in his newly slimmed state.

The popularity of Mr. Banting's diet lasted only a few years. It was later replaced by other diets, such as Fletcherism (slow eating) and Phtoline (the use of a purgative), to name just a few. Unlike fleetingingly popular previous diets, though, the Atkins diet has continued to grow in acceptance, both by the medical community and the general population. Several other plans have also been published similarly promoting low-carbohydrate intake, such as the South Beach Diet, Sugar Busters, the Carbohydrate Addict, the Zone, and Protein Power. Each emphasizes the need to restrict carbohydrates in the diet, but individual authors offer a slightly different approach to the original Atkins concept.

As popular and effective as these diets are, many low-carb enthusiasts find it difficult to completely give up all the wonderfully satisfying foods and beverages they enjoyed in the past. Unfortunately, a sweet tooth can't be extracted by the dentist. One of the ways many of us enjoyed satisfying our sugar-loving incisors in 2005 B.C. (Before Carbs) was with a rich and syrupy smoothie. These mellow concoctions, made from the tantalizing union of fruit and fruit juice, are easy to prepare, inherently flavorful, and even provide significant health benefits. However, as tasty and healthful as your favorite traditional smoothies may be, they are almost certainly not carb-friendly. Unfortunately, traditional smoothie ingredients such as fruits, fruit juice, most yogurts, ice cream, and other dairy products contain unacceptably high amounts of carbohydrates.

The good news is that I have overcome this obstacle. Today, with the amazing low-carb recipes found in this book, you can actually splurge on a flavorful smoothie without losing ground in the battle of the bulge. Get ready to discover in these pages that smoothies, when properly prepared, can be reinvented as a low-carb indulgence that is sweet and satisfying. By simply choosing only carb-friendly fruit, substituting zero- or low-carb ingredients, and adding a variety of sugar-free flavor enhancements, you can create a wonder-in-a-glass that is low-carb legal, yet amazingly rewarding in taste.

Adding smaller servings of fruit to smoothies is one strategy to keep the carb count at bay. To compensate for the diminished fruit content, a variety of carb-friendly protein powders is recommended to add both thickness and extra nutrition. Be aware, however, that there is a wide variance in the carb count among the different brands of protein powders, and this often suggests the use of one protein powder over another in a given recipe. For instance, I suggest using Zone Perfect protein powder in some smoothie recipes because it has 0 grams of carbohydrates and adds just the right amount of bulk, whereas I have included Amplify by Release dietary supplement in other recipes for its high protein content, even at the expense of a few more carbs. Please don't hesitate to substitute any of your favorite protein powders, even if only because it is what's readily available in your pantry or in the health section of your local supermarket.

Low-Carb Smoothies appropriately begins with a chapter entitled, "The Skinny on Low-Carb Diets: What's It All About?" This section starts with definitions of important terms such as carbohydrates and related topics including insulin, ketones, and glycogen. The accompanying discussion in this chapter will help you understand the philosophy behind the low-carb diet. If you are already following one of the low-carb diets or have reached your target weight, this may not be entirely new information. However, if you are curious about the diet or are contemplating trying it, my goal is to present enough basic information to provide a foundation that can be built upon by more in-depth discussions of the concept by scientists, nutritionists, and other experts in this area.

In chapter 2, "Fruit for Thought: Low-Carb Smoothie Ingredients," you will discover the secrets of selecting and preparing the best carb-friendly fruits. Chapter 3, "Getting up to Speed: All You'll Ever Need to Know to Prepare a Low-Carb Smoothie," will help you become more familiar with the techniques and essential equipment you'll need in order to transform your kitchen into an eternal spring of low-carb smoothies. You will discover a host of helpful tips that will enable you to elevate every low-carb smoothie masterpiece you prepare to the absolute pinnacle of frosty elation.

As you browse through the following chapters containing smoothie recipes, you will find that each one is divided into two sections: one featuring Low-Carb Smoothies and the other, Ultra Low-Carb Smoothies. Using chapter 4, "Simple Pleasures," as an example, you'll find that smoothies in the Low-Carb Smoothies section contain 10 grams of carbohydrates or less, while those in Ultra Low-Carb Smoothies have 6 grams of carbohydrates or less. In each chapter, this division will enable you to choose the recipes that best fit your diet plan, depending on how carb-stingy it is or may become. I chose those ingredients that had the absolute lowest carbohydrate count.

Be aware that different brands of similar low-carb products can actually vary significantly in true carbohydrate content. For example, I found that ½ cup of 4% milk fat cottage cheese can range from 3 to 5 grams of carbohydrates, depending on the manufacturer. Likewise, KĒTO brand instant sugar-free pudding has fewer carbs than the usual sugar-free variety readily available in supermarkets (you can find a list of suggested low-carb products in chapter 8, "Mail-Order and Online Shopping," on page 207).

Another thing to consider is the discrepancy between net carbs (or *effective* or *impact* carbs) and total carbs. For example, the nutritional label found on the back of a gallon of low-carb ice cream may say it contains 20 grams of total carbohydrates per serving, whereas the label found on the front of the carton may claim that the same serving has only 3 "net carbs." How can this be? According to the manufacturer, in this case only 3 carbohydrate grams actually raise the blood sugar level while the remaining 17, derived from sources such as fiber, sugar alcohol, and glycerin, have only a *minimal impact*. Until the FDA approves of labeling that makes a distinction between net and total carbs, I remain hesitant about purchasing products that claim to have a low net carb content but actually have a relatively high total carb count. In this book, only the total carb count is considered in each recipe.

With these principles in mind, you'll be delighted to find three chapters devoted to mouthwatering low-carb smoothie recipes that will appeal to all smoothie enthusiasts. For example, you'll be tempted by more than forty recipes in chapter 4, "Simple Pleasures: Basic Low-Carb Favorites." These delectable smoothies, made with a variety of low-carb ingredients but containing few fortifying ingredients, are among the lowest in carbohydrate content. Some of my favorite creations are Carb Talk, made with French vanilla–flavored AdvantEdge Carb Control shake, raspberry yogurt, raspberries, and strawberries, and Almond Chocolate E-Carbs, made with a low-carb chocolate beverage, strawberries, and raspberries, topped off with almond and chocolate syrups. Both are a low-carb fantasy come true.

The next chapter, "Frosty and Fortified: Pumped-Up Smoothies for Your Health," contains more than forty recipes made with additional healthful ingredients such as flax or soybean products for their health-enhancing properties and protein supplements to bring each glassful closer to meal replacement status. Each smoothie in this chapter is a celebration of well-being that will also satisfy the snackaholic in you. If you're looking for a way to add more flax to your low-carb diet, imagine sipping a strawful of Raspberry Flax, Not Fiction, a prescription in a glass that is made with soy milk, flaxseed oil, and raspberries. On the other hand, if you're looking for a quick energy boost, consider mixing up a batch of Berry Fuel-Efficient Carbs, a protein powder–enriched blend made with French vanilla–flavored Advant-Edge Carb Control shake, blueberries, and raspberries.

The frosty creations in chapter 6, "Maintenance Low-Carb Smoothies: Now That You've Taken It Off, Keep It Off!," are designed to appeal to those of you who have successfully reached your target weight and simply want to maintain it. While it remains important to avoid foods that are truly not carb-friendly, it may be possible to add just a few more carbs to your daily meal plan at this stage. In keeping with this slight shift in your low-carb plan, you will note that the definition of Ultra Low-Carb and Low-Carb in this chapter have been slightly ratcheted up to accommodate the more liberal carb intake that successful dieters earn. With just a few more carbs, you'll discover that these wonderful creations are a perfect snack to indulge in when you are tempted to "fall off the wagon."

Finally, chapter 7, "The Garnish Factor: How to Embellish a Low-Carb Smoothie," contains recipes for edible garnishes that will enable you to transform any of your favorite low-carb smoothie creations into a visually striking and impressive presentation without adding too many extra carbs.

The recipes featured in this book will convince you that smoothies can easily be transformed from fattening to flattering. Whether you indulge while in the Zone or on a South Beach, you're due for some entirely legal satisfaction in a glass!

The Skinny on Low-Carb Diets

What's It All About?

If you wish to grow thinner,
diminish your dinner.

—H. S. LEIGH

UNDERSTANDING THE METABOLIC AND NUTRI-
tional principles behind the low-carbohydrate diet is
not rocket science, but without an adequate discussion outlined in simple terms it can seem that way.
There are only a few simple definitions that you
need to familiarize yourself with in order to clearly
understand the scientific theory behind the diet
and how it allows you to lose weight in an easy and
healthful way. So, before delving into the explana-
tion, let's define those terms that will set you on
the pathway to becoming a first-class carbomeister.

- **Calorie**   Officially a measure of heat, a calorie,
  in dietary terms, is a measure of the amount of

energy the body can derive from a particular food. The more calories provided by a foodstuff, the longer it will take the body to "burn up" that nutrient.

- **Carbohydrate**   Carbohydrates are one of three major nutrient groups that provide energy for the body, the other two being protein and fat. All carbohydrates are composed of single sugars or strings of sugar bound together. Single sugars, such as table sugar (sucrose), fruit sugar (fructose), and dairy sugar (lactose), are referred to as simple carbohydrates. Plants bind excessive sugars together, resulting in complex carbohydrates, often referred to as starches. Most complex carbohydrates, such as potato starch or wheat flour, are edible and digestible, but some, such as cellulose (from celery), cannot be digested.

- **Glucose**   Glucose (also known as dextrose) is a simple sugar found in fruits and honey. It is also the form of sugar that circulates in the human bloodstream. The blood level of glucose is the major stimulus for insulin secretion from the pancreas.

- **Glycogen**   Glycogen is the form in which the body stores excess glucose in the liver and muscles. It is essentially composed of a number of glucose molecules strung together. Glycogen is an energy storehouse for the body, and when needed, it can be broken down into glucose and released from its storage sites.

- **Glucagon**   Glucagon is one of two major hormones produced by the pancreas (the other is insulin). When the blood sugar level is low, glucagon is released and acts to stimulate the liver to break down its stored glycogen into glucose and release it into the bloodstream. This hormone also promotes the breakdown of protein and fat to produce energy when blood glucose is not at an adequate level for the body's needs.

- **Glycemic Index** The glycemic index of a carbohydrate-containing food is a measure of the degree it raises your blood sugar after it is eaten. For example, white bread raises blood sugar higher and faster than apples, so its glycemic index is high, while apples get a low glycemic index rating.

- **Insulin** Insulin is one of two major hormones produced by the pancreas (the other is glucagon). It is released by the pancreas when the blood glucose rises and then helps transfer glucose into cells where it can be used as a source of energy. In fatty tissue, insulin promotes the conversion of excess glucose to fat, and in the liver it causes excess glucose to be stored as glycogen. In muscle, it promotes the entry of amino acids, the building blocks of protein. Diabetes is due to inadequate production of insulin, reduced sensitivity to its effect, or both. When insulin secretion is excessive, this hormone can elevate cholesterol levels and inhibit the breakdown of previously stored fat.

- **Ketones** Ketones are chemicals that result from the breakdown of fat that occurs when the body does not have enough glucose for energy production and the liver's store of glycogen has been used up. Although there are always some ketones circulating in the blood-stream, fasting or a very low-carbohydrate diet increases the amount of these substances, creating a condition referred to as *ketosis*.

With these definitions in mind, how does the low-carbohydrate diet work? In the simplest terms, the body's response to a carbohydrate meal is to se-crete insulin, while at the same time suppressing release of the other pancreatic hormone, glucagon. As we age, excessive insulin secretion can occur in response to even ordinary amounts of carbohy-drates in the diet because of insulin resistance, a condition in which our cells respond subnormally to the hormone, requiring the pancreas to secrete more of it just to achieve a normal effect. One of the basic underlying principles of the low-carbohydrate diet is that insulin (especially exces-sive insulin) has potentially negative health effects, while the opposite is true for glucagon. After a high-carbohydrate meal, insulin tries to store the excess glucose derived from the meal as glycogen in the liver and muscles. Because this storage capacity is limited and easily saturated, insulin next turns to fat as a storage vehicle for the re-maining glucose. Not only does excess insulin pro-mote the deposition of fat in this way, it may also have other negative health effects, such as eleva-tion of blood cholesterol and retention of fluid and salt.

Now that you understand the metabolic and nutritional principles behind the low-carbohydrate diet, you are ready to become a convert to this exciting way of dieting, or, if you're already con-verted, to exclaim a few hallelujahs. The common thread running through all low-carb diets is the requirement to restrict the daily consumption of all foods that are high in carbohydrates. It sounds simple, but this may be a challenging feat for many of us to accomplish, and giving up traditionally high-carb foods that have always been a source of enjoyment and satisfaction can be a major stumbling block. Enter *Low-Carb Smoothies*. Now the promise of being able to enjoy some of the same treats that you savored in the pre-carb era can help you make the leap to a true low-carb lifestyle.

· 2 ·

Fruit for Thought

Low-Carb Smoothie Ingredients

Time flies like an arrow.
Fruit flies like a banana.

—GROUCHO MARX

FRESH FRUIT IS AN IMPORTANT COMPONENT of most smoothies. While many of these delectable bundles of vitamins have a high carbohydrate count, a wide variety of more carb-friendly orchard bounty remains available for use on your mission to create the perfect low-carb smoothie. The objective of this chapter is to acquaint you with these carb-friendly fruits and to guide you in choosing, storing, and preparing them. To begin with, it is important to realize that choosing fruit that is smoothie-ready can be very deceptive, especially if your choice is based on appearance alone. At first glance, a peach may look ripe simply because of its rich color. There are, however, a number of other less obvious but equally important attributes to consider. You should attempt to determine whether the fruit has a fresh aroma, how heavy or dense it is, and whether it is firm yet yields slightly to gentle pressure. These characteristics are often more important than the fruit's color. The good news is that once you become a fruit connoisseur, you will find that it's actually quite easy to determine whether fruit is ripe.

I am certain that as you become more familiar with the wide array of fruit available, you will delight in the excitement of including it in this new generation of delicious smoothies. As you navigate the aisles of your favorite farmer's market or produce department, I hope you find the following information useful in your quest for the best nature has to offer.

APPLE

Apples are believed to have originated in Central Asia and the Caucasus. They have been cultivated since prehistoric times. They were brought to the United States at the beginning of the seventeenth century and later to Africa and Australia. Today, more than a hundred varieties of apples are commercially grown in the United States.

Apples, whether red, green, or yellow, all have a firm, crisp flesh. They are a rich source of fiber. Some apples have a sweet flavor with a hint of tartness, while others are less sweet and more tart. Most apples are delicious when made into a smoothie, but your flavor preference will determine the best variety for you. Apples are available year-round, but are at their peak in October and November.

Selection

When choosing an apple, look for one that is firm and crisp with a smooth, tight skin. Most important, the apple should have a sweet-smelling aroma. Avoid any apple that has a bruised or blemished skin. Buy the organic variety whenever possible. Most nonorganic apples are heavily sprayed with pesticides and later waxed to preserve them and keep them looking fresh. This can affect the taste, not to mention your health. Should you find a worm in an organic apple, simply remove the unwelcome visitor when you cut the apple, thereby removing any health or aesthetic concerns. Wash all apples in cool water and dry them well before cutting. Uncut apples can be stored in the crisper bin of the refrigerator for up to six weeks if they are kept separate from other fruits and vegetables.

APRICOT

The apricot is a round or oblong fruit measuring about two inches in diameter with skin and flesh that are golden orange in color. It is a very sweet and juicy fruit with a single, smooth stone. The apricot is native to North China and was known to be a food source as early as 2200 B.C. Apricots are available from May through July.

Selection

When choosing apricots, look for those that are well colored, plump, and fairly firm but yield slightly when gently pressed. An apricot that is soft to the touch and juicy is fully ripe and should be eaten or used in a smoothie right away. If an apricot is hard, it can be placed in a brown paper bag and allowed to ripen at room temperature for a day or two. Avoid apricots that are green in color because they will not ripen or be good for consumption. Refrigerate ripe apricots in the crisper bin of the refrigerator for up to a week. Wash them in cool water just before using them.

BANANA

The banana has been around for so long that according to Hindu legend, it was actually the forbidden fruit of the Garden of Eden. It is also believed that the banana was widely cultivated throughout Asia and Oceania before recorded history and that the Spanish colonists introduced banana shoots to the New World in 1516.

Bananas have a high glycemic level and should be avoided when following a low-carb diet. For those who have achieved their weight-loss goal, adding a banana to one's diet is a healthy alternative. Bananas are available year-round.

Selection

Bananas are picked when they are green and sweeten as they ripen. When choosing a banana, look for one that is completely yellow. The riper a banana, or the more yellow its skin, the sweeter it is. Bananas that are yellow but have green tips and green necks or that are all yellow except for light green necks are also ready to eat. Green bananas will ripen at room temperature in two or three days. Alternatively, they can be placed in a brown paper bag to accelerate the ripening process. If a tomato or apple is added to the bag, the bananas will ripen even faster because fruit cells produce a colorless gas called ethylene, which stimulates ripening in many fruits and some vegetables. Ripe bananas can be stored at room temperature or in the refrigerator for a couple of days.

BLACKBERRY

The blackberry is a small black, blue, or dark red berry that grows on thorny bushes (brambles).

These berries are oblong in shape and grow up to one inch in length. The United States is the world's dominant producer of blackberries. Blackberries are at their peak in flavor and availability from June through September, but may still be found in some supermarkets from November on into April.

Selection

When choosing blackberries, look for ones that are plump and solid with full color and a bright, fresh appearance. Place them in a shallow container to prevent the berries on top from crushing those on the bottom. Cover the container and store it in the crisper bin of the refrigerator for one to two days. Wash blackberries in cool water just before you are ready to use them.

BLUEBERRY

Native to North America, the blueberry has the distinction of being the second most popular berry in the United States. It has been around for thousands of years, but was not cultivated until the turn of the twentieth century. Today, 95 percent of the world's commercial crop of blueberries is grown in the United States. Blueberries are at their peak in flavor from mid-April to late September. They are available in the southern states first and gradually move north as the season progresses.

Selection

When choosing blueberries, look for those that are plump and firm with a dark blue color and a silvery bloom. The bloom on blueberries is the dusty powder that protects them from the sun; it does not rinse off. Avoid any berries that appear to be dull because this may indicate that the fruit is old.

Blueberries should be prepared in the same way as blackberries, washed just prior to use, but they can be stored unwashed for a longer time in the crisper bin of the refrigerator, from three to five days.

KIWIFRUIT

The kiwifruit, about the size of a plum, grows on a vine. It has a brown fuzzy skin and a luscious sweet-and-sour emerald green pulp that surrounds a cluster of black seeds. Kiwifruit originated in the 1600s in the Yangtze River valley in China, where it was called Yangtao. In 1906, Yangtao seeds were sent to New Zealand, where the fruit was re-named the Chinese gooseberry. In 1962, the Chinese gooseberry was shipped to the United States, where it was again renamed the kiwifruit in honor of New Zealand's famous national bird. Kiwifruit are at their peak from June to October.

Selection

When choosing a kiwifruit, look for one that is light brown, has a sweet aroma, and is firm yet will give slightly when pressed. Kiwifruit will ripen at room temperature in three to five days. Kiwifruit can also be placed in a brown paper bag along with an apple or banana to speed the ripening process. Store ripe kiwifruit in the crisper bin of the refrigerator for up to three weeks.

ORANGE

Fresh oranges are widely grown in Florida, California, and Arizona and are available all year long. The two major varieties are the Valencia and navel. Two other varieties grown in the Western states are the Cara Cara and Moro (similar to the blood orange). Moros are available from December through May and Cara Cara from late December through March.

Selection

When selecting an orange, look for one that is heavy for its size and firm. Avoid oranges with a bruised skin, indicating possible fermentation, as well as those with a loose skin, suggesting they may be dry inside. Although oranges can be stored at room temperature for a few days, their flavor is best when they are kept refrigerated for up to two weeks.

PEACH and NECTARINE

Grown since prehistoric times, peaches were first cultivated in China. They were later introduced into Europe and Persia. It is believed that the Spaniards brought peaches to North, Central, and South America. Spanish missionaries planted the first peach trees in California.

Numerous varieties of peaches are available, and they are broken down into rough classifications. One type of peach is the freestone, so named because the pit separates easily from the peach. Another variety is the clingstone, in which the pit is firmly attached to the fruit. The freestone is the peach most often found in supermarkets because it is easy to eat, while clingstones are frequently canned.

The nectarine is a smooth-skinned variety of the peach.

Peaches and nectarines are ripe in the summer months and are at their peak in taste in August.

Selection

When picking peaches, look for ones that are relatively firm with a fuzzy, creamy yellow skin and a sweet aroma. The pink blush on the peach indicates its variety, not its ripeness. Avoid peaches with a wrinkled skin or those that are soft or blemished. A ripe peach should yield gently when touched. To ripen peaches, keep them at room temperature and out of direct sunlight until the skin yields slightly to the touch. Once they are ripe, store them in a single layer in the crisper bin of the refrigerator for up to five days. Wash peaches in cool water just before you are ready to use them.

When choosing nectarines, look for those with bright red markings over a yellow skin. Avoid any with a wrinkled skin or those that are soft and bruised. The nectarine should yield gently to the touch and have a sweet aroma. To ripen nectarines, place them in a brown paper bag and keep them at room temperature. Once they are ripe, store them in a single layer in the crisper bin of the refrigerator for up to a week. Wash nectarines in cool water just before you are ready to use them.

RASPBERRY

It is believed that red raspberries spread all over Europe and Asia in prehistoric times. Because they were so plentiful and delicious growing wild, it was not until the 1600s that raspberries were cultivated in Europe. Those that are cultivated in North America originate from two groups: the wild red raspberry, native to Europe, and the red variety, native to northeastern America.

Selection

When choosing raspberries, it is always best to buy them when they are in season—usually starting in late June and lasting four to six weeks. If you are fortunate enough to live near a berry farm, take advantage of it by visiting at the beginning of the season to get the best pick. Select berries that are large and plump, bright, shiny, uniform in color, and free of mold. Avoid any that are mushy. Before refrigerating raspberries, carefully go through the batch and discard any that show signs of spoilage. Place the raspberries in a shallow container to prevent the berries on top from crushing those on the bottom. Cover the container and store it in the crisper bin of the refrigerator for one to two days. Wash raspberries in cool water just before you are ready to use them.

STRAWBERRY

Strawberries date as far back as 2,200 years. They are known to have grown wild in Italy in the third century, and by 1588, they were discovered in Virginia by the first European settlers. Local Indians cultivated the strawberry as early as the mid-1600s, and by the middle of the nineteenth century, this fruit was widely grown in many parts of North America.

The strawberry grows in groups of three on the stem of a plant that is very low to the ground. As the fruit ripens, it changes from greenish white in color to a lush flame red. The strawberry does not have a skin but is actually covered by hundreds of tiny seeds.

Selection

The best time to buy strawberries is in June and July when they are at their peak of juicy freshness. As with raspberries, if you are lucky enough to live near a strawberry farm, a pick-your-own day trip is a wonderful family outing as well as an excellent way to get the very best of the crop. Look for plump, firm, and deep-colored fruit with a bright green cap and a sweet strawberry aroma. Strawberries can be stored in a single layer in the crisper bin of the refrigerator for up to two days. Wash them with their caps in cool water just before you are ready to use them.

TANGERINE

Tangerines, also known as Mandarins, are a close cousin of the orange. Native to Southeastern Asia, they have been widely cultivated in orange-growing regions of the world. While tangerines resemble an orange, they are smaller in size and oblong in shape but can be slightly flat on each end. Another variety of the tangerine is the clementine, sometimes called an Algerian tangerine. Clementines are a cross between a Mandarin orange and a Seville orange and are usually seedless. Because all tangerines have a loose, puffy skin, these sweet juicy fruits peel easily and their sections can be readily separated.

Selection

Choose tangerines that have a deep, glossy orange skin and are heavy for their size. Tangerines are usually ripe and ready to eat when you buy them, but they can be left on the kitchen counter for up to one week at a cool room temperature or stored in the crisper bin of the refrigerator away from vegetables for up to two weeks.

FREEZING FRUIT

Because fruit is so perishable, you may want to freeze some while it is in season to store for later use. By purchasing an ample quantity to freeze, you can be certain of having on hand a supply of any fruit you know will not be available after a certain date when you need it to prepare one of your favorite low-carb smoothies. Also, there may be times when already ripened fruit isn't needed immediately. Freezing prevents overripening and allows it to be utilized at a later time.

To make a low-carb smoothie with the optimal consistency, it is important that you freeze for thirty minutes or more any fresh fruit you use. Using partially frozen fruit also helps maintain your smoothie at an ideal icy-cold temperature.

Whether you are freezing fruit for immediate use or for storage, the basic preparation is identical.

- When you are ready to freeze **apricots** (which should be cut in half with their stones removed) or **berries**, place them in a colander and rinse them with a gentle stream of cool water. Pat them dry with a paper towel.

- To freeze a **peach** or **nectarine** (remove its stone), wash it and cut it into small pieces.

- To freeze a **banana** or **kiwifruit**, remove its skin and either slice it or freeze it whole and then slice it later, before use.

- Before freezing **oranges** and **tangerines**, remove the peel and pith, break each into segments, and remove any seeds.

- To prepare **apples** for freezing, remove their peels and seeds before cubing.

Place the prepared fruit on a baking sheet lined with freezer paper, plastic-coated side facing up to prevent it from sticking to the surface. (In a pinch, wax paper or parchment paper can be used instead.) If you are storing the fruit to use at a later date, transfer it to an airtight plastic bag. Label the contents, mark the date on the bag, and freeze the fruit for up to two weeks. Most fruit can be kept in the freezer this long without a loss of flavor. If you are preparing the fruit for immediate use, freeze it for at least thirty minutes, after which time it will be ready to add to your other smoothie ingredients.

HOW MUCH FRUIT SHOULD I BUY?

To determine how much fruit you will need to make a smoothie, consult the list below for an estimate of the quantity of fruit (in number of cups) you'll actually end up with once the skin, hull, seeds, pit, and core are removed. You can use the average weight per individual fruit provided in the table, or to be more precise, you can weigh the fruit, using the supermarket scale, before you purchase it.

FRUIT	How Much to Buy	Average Weight	Number of Cups
Apple	1 medium	6 ounces	1 cup
Apricots	3	8 ounces	1 cup
Banana	1 large	10 ounces	1 cup
Blackberries	1/2 pint	6 ounces	1 1/4 cups
Blueberries	1/2 pint	8 ounces	1 cup
Kiwifruit	3	8 ounces	1 cup
Nectarine	1 medium	8 ounces	1 cup
Orange	1 medium	10 ounces	1 cup
Peach	1 medium	8 ounces	1 cup
Raspberries	1 box	6 ounces	1 1/4 cups
Strawberries	7 to 8 medium	6 ounces	1 cup
Tangerine	1 small	5 ounces	1/2 cup

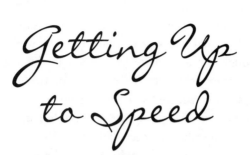

· 3 ·

Getting Up to Speed

All You'll Ever Need to Know to Prepare a Low-Carb Smoothie

*In department stores,
so much kitchen equipment is bought
indiscriminately by people who just
come in for men's underwear.*

—JULIA CHILD

ASIDE FROM FABULOUS TASTE, A UNIQUE ATTRAC-
tion of smoothies is that they are unbelievably
quick and easy to prepare. With very little effort,
you can enjoy a satisfying and richly flavored drink
within minutes. With such an unbeatable combination of good taste and ease of preparation, it is no
wonder smoothies have quickly become one of the
most popular culinary rages of our era.

You don't need to have an extensive array of
equipment in your kitchen to prepare a low-carb
smoothie. In fact, all you need is a modest number
of essential tools: a sharp knife for prepping fruit,
measuring spoons and cups, a rubber spatula to
remove every last drop from the blender, airtight

freezer bags for storing freshly cut fruit in the freezer, and, of course, the essential blender (or food processor).

You might want to consider, in addition, a few optional items of equipment. As you glance through the garnish recipes found in this cookbook, you will note the mention of two useful tools not considered standard kitchen equipment. The first, a silicone mat, is a reusable laminated food-grade silicone sheet with a nonstick surface that is used to line a baking sheet. The second, a mandoline slicer, is a handheld kitchen implement containing a variety of cartridge blades that perform precision cutting of foods in several modes such as very thick, very thin, and julienne, just to mention a few. Again, these are very helpful items, but neither is an absolute necessity.

Finally, although a food processor can be used to make a smoothie, most smoothie experts would agree that a blender is definitely the preferred appliance. Unlike the blender container, the food processor bowl is wide and low, causing food to be sent sideways rather than upward by the spinning blade. This motion results in food striking the sides of the container, with less incorporation of air than the upward motion produced by a blender. Moreover, when a food processor is used to purée fruit and ice, it often leaves small chunks of ice behind, as opposed to a blender, which breaks up the ice and fruit into tiny particles. Still, if a food processor is all you have, it should do fine. Your smoothies just won't be as perfect.

THE BLENDER

The blender is the most important piece of kitchen equipment when it comes to making a proper smoothie. Credit for the invention of this indis-pensable appliance goes to Stephen J. Poplawski, who, in 1922, first conceived of placing a spinning blade at the bottom of a glass container. By 1935, Fred Waring and Frederick Osius had made significant improvements on the original design and began marketing the Waring Blender. The rest is history.

A blender basically consists of a tall and narrow stainless steel, plastic, or glass food container fitted with metal blades at the bottom. These blades usually have four cutting edges placed on two or four planes allowing for the ingredients in the container to hit multiple cutting surfaces. The rapidly spinning blades cause an upward motion, creating a vortex in the container that allows for the incorporation of more air in the final product, giving it a smoother consistency.

When selecting a blender, you should assess certain basic qualities, including its durability, ease of operation and cleaning, capacity, and noise production. With such a wide variety of blenders from which to choose, I hope the following information will help you narrow your choice.

- Blender containers typically come in two sizes: thirty-two ounces and forty ounces. If you will routinely be preparing smoothies for more than two people, choose the larger one.

- Blender motors come in different sizes. Those with 290-watt motors are adequate for most blending jobs but not optimal for smoothies. Those with 330- to 400-watt motors, considered to be of professional caliber, are excellent for crushing ice, a very important feature for creating the best smoothies.

- Blenders can be found with a variety of blade speed options, ranging from two speeds (high and low) to multiple (between five and fourteen) speeds. Variable-speed models provide more options, such as the ability to liquefy and whip.

- The blender should have a removable bottom for ease of cleaning.

- Container lids should have a secondary lid that can be easily removed. This allows for the addition of ingredients while the blender is turned on.

- Avoid plastic container jars because they become scratched over time and do not wash well in the dishwasher.

Recently, new blenders specifically designed for making smoothies have become available. One whirring wizard, called the Smoothie Elite (by Back to Basics), has several features, including a custom stir stick to break up the air pockets, an ice-crunching blade that assures consistent smoothie texture, and a convenient spigot at the bottom of the container that serves up the finished product.

Once you have decided on the features you would like in a blender, I encourage you to visit several appliance or department stores and personally view the various models available. The salesclerk should be able to provide you with information to further help you in making the best decision.

The Internet is another resource for gleaning valuable information. Many of the companies that manufacture these appliances have very informative sites describing their individual product, and some also provide a phone number so you can speak to a representative. Finally, *Consumer Reports* and similar publications provide comparison quality ratings of a variety of blenders.

HELPFUL TECHNIQUES

Now that the blender (or food processor) has taken its rightful place, center stage on your countertop, it is time to rev it up and make a low-carb smoothie. I hope you found equipping your kitchen with the necessary tools to make smoothies a relatively easy process. You will be pleased to learn that mastering the techniques required to prepare them is no more difficult. In fact, preparing a smoothie may be one of the most uncomplicated tasks you will ever perform in your kitchen. All you have to do is simply place the appropriate smoothie ingredients in a blender and you will end up with a wonderfully delicious final product. However, for those who want to create the "truly perfect" low-carb smoothie, I have discovered a few additional techniques that will help you reach that lofty goal.

- To get the most delicious fruit, buy it when it is in season and at its peak in flavor.

- Before freezing fruit, wash and dry it, then follow the preparation instructions given in the previous chapter.

- Store-bought individually frozen fruit can be substituted for fresh frozen fruit, but it should be used within six months of the purchase date. Avoid using frozen fruit that is packaged in sweetened syrup.

- To be certain that you have a supply of your favorite seasonal fruits, stock up before they are no longer available for purchase. Although fruits have the most flavor when they are kept frozen for only one to two weeks, they can be kept in the freezer for a slightly longer amount of time and still be edible.

- When adding ingredients to a blender, always add the liquid first, then the frozen fruit, and the ice cream last.

- If the fruit you have frozen becomes clumped together, gently pound it within the sealed bag with a mallet or blunt object until the pieces separate.

- If the smoothie is too thin, add more fruit. Conversely, if the smoothie is too thick, add more of your favorite low-carb beverage.

· 4 ·

Simple Pleasures

Basic Low-Carb Favorites

———

The difference between try and
triumph is just a little umph!

—Marvin Phillips

SMOOTHIES ARE ONE OF THE MOST CELEBRATED
and refreshing taste treats to have emerged in
recent years. The cool creations described in this
chapter, made with a simple combination of carb-
friendly fruits and a variety of low-carb shake
mixes, soft drinks, and flavor enhancers, are a delicious low-carb alternative to the traditional high-
carb variety that sinfully resemble malts, milk
shakes, or blizzards. It is important to realize that
the carb count in many ordinary smoothies can be
deceptively high unless they have been prepared
with careful attention to the ingredients used. One
example of the techniques employed in this book
to avoid this mega-carbohydrate trap is to use
strawberries and raspberries frequently to provide
just the right amount of sweetness and texture,
while still remaining faithful to the low-carb spirit.

The resulting low-carb pleasures are not only delicious, they deserve at least one more kudo: With every swallow you are on your way to fulfilling the American Cancer Institute's recommendation to include at least two to three servings of fruit in your diet each day.

As you glance through this chapter, you will be impressed with the great variety of low-carb smoothies that can easily be created with a combination of carb-friendly fruits, and I feel confident that you will be delighted with the flavorful and satisfying result that each recipe provides. Be ready to be impressed when you try Strawberry Scorn on the Carb, a refreshing smoothie featuring strawberries blended with a low-carb dairy beverage, banana syrup, and vanilla-flavored Atkins shake mix. If you're a raspberry devotee, then you will be thrilled with the taste of Raspberry Carb Shark, a delicious blend of raspberries, raspberry syrup, low-carb dairy beverage, and raspberry-flavored ice cubes.

Keep in mind that a little experimentation with the suggested ingredients is allowed depending on your taste or what is readily available in your pantry. For example, you will notice that one of the key flavor enhancers in many low-carb smoothies is a sugar-free syrup. While I may suggest using strawberry syrup in a smoothie made with strawberries and raspberries, feel free to experiment with a raspberry, blueberry, or even pineapple syrup instead. Don't hold back; just dive in and create your own signature smoothies. You'll be amazed at how a few spins of your blender can liberate you from low-carb boredom.

Simple Pleasures

ULTRA LOW-CARB SMOOTHIES

These smoothies
have *6* grams
of carbohydrates
or less.

Almond Chocolate E-Carbs

Make someone's day by e-mailing this tantalizing low-carb recipe along with a special greeting.

1 SERVING

¼ cup chocolate Carb Countdown (or favorite low-carb) dairy beverage

2 tablespoons creamy vanilla–flavored Atkins Advantage (or favorite low-carb) ready-to-drink shake

2 tablespoons sugar-free almond syrup

2 tablespoons sugar-free chocolate syrup

¼ cup partially frozen raspberries

¼ cup partially frozen diced strawberries

Place all the ingredients in a blender container in the order listed. Place the cover on the container. Turn on the blender and process by pressing the pulse button, while on the lowest blade-speed setting, until the ingredients are mostly blended. Continue mixing without the pulse function by pressing the highest blade-speed setting button until the mixture is smooth (it may be necessary to turn off the blender periodically and stir the mixture with a spoon, working from the bottom up). Turn off the blender. Pour the smoothie into a glass and garnish with a Chocolate-Dipped Strawberry (page 196), if desired.

Anne of Lean Gables

Now that you've adopted the habit of eating low-carb foods, this flavorful low-carb strawberry and orange blend will make you feel like you're cheating—but you're not. This one is for keeps.

1 SERVING

6 to 8 tablespoons diet orange soda
2 tablespoons sugar-free cherry syrup
6 tablespoons partially frozen diced strawberries
2 tablespoons partially frozen diced orange
1 scoop vanilla-flavored Atkins (or favorite low-carb) shake mix
½ teaspoon sugar-free orange Jell-O powder
¼ to ½ teaspoon ground cinnamon, or to taste

Place all the ingredients in a blender container in the order listed. Place the cover on the container. Turn on the blender and process by pressing the pulse button, while on the lowest blade-speed setting, until the ingredients are mostly blended. Continue mixing without the pulse function by pressing the highest blade-speed setting button until the mixture is smooth (it may be necessary to turn off the blender periodically and stir the mixture with a spoon, working from the bottom up). Turn off the blender. Pour the smoothie into a glass and garnish the rim with an Orange Wheel (page 200), if desired.

Berry Manilow

If you're "ready to take a chance again" with a new kind of low-carb taste treat, then "this one's for you." Made with raspberries and strawberries, "it's a miracle" how a low-carb smoothie can taste this good.

1 SERVING

½ cup Carb Countdown (or favorite low-carb) dairy beverage
2 tablespoons sugar-free raspberry syrup
¼ cup partially frozen raspberries
¼ cup partially frozen diced strawberries
½ cup crushed frozen Minute Maid Light mango tropical (or favorite low-carb) fruit drink cubes
½ teaspoon sugar-free raspberry Jell-O powder

Place all the ingredients in a blender container in the order listed. Place the cover on the container. Turn on the blender and process by pressing the pulse button, while on the lowest blade-speed setting, until the ingredients are mostly blended. Continue mixing without the pulse function by pressing the highest blade-speed setting button until the mixture is smooth (it may be necessary to turn off the blender periodically and stir the mixture with a spoon, working from the bottom up). Turn off the blender. Pour the smoothie into a glass and garnish the rim with a Strawberry Fan (page 205), if desired.

Berry Slim Odds

Chances are you're craving refreshment that's both satisfying and delicious. Well, I bet you'll fall in love with this flavorful strawberry smoothie after one sip.

1 SERVING

4 to 6 tablespoons raspberry ice (or favorite flavor) Crystal Light soft drink
2 tablespoons sugar-free cherry syrup
$\frac{1}{2}$ cup partially frozen diced strawberries
1 teaspoon sugar-free strawberry Jell-O powder
$\frac{1}{2}$ cup crushed frozen Minute Maid Light raspberry passion (or favorite low-carb) fruit drink cubes

Place all the ingredients in a blender container in the order listed. Place the cover on the container. Turn on the blender and process by pressing the pulse button, while on the lowest blade-speed setting, until the ingredients are mostly blended. Continue mixing without the pulse function by pressing the highest blade-speed setting button until the mixture is smooth (it may be necessary to turn off the blender periodically and stir the mixture with a spoon, working from the bottom up). Turn off the blender. Pour the smoothie into a glass and garnish with Berries on a Skewer (page 189), if desired.

Blue(berry)s Brothers

If you feel like you've been a prisoner to a bland low-carb regimen, then don a pair of dark sunglasses and get ready to sample this refreshingly sweet blueberry smoothie.

1 SERVING

4 to 6 tablespoons diet cherry soda
2 tablespoons sugar-free cherry syrup
6 tablespoons partially frozen blueberries
1 scoop Zone Perfect (or favorite low-carb) protein powder
1 teaspoon sugar-free cherry Jell-O powder

Place all the ingredients in a blender container in the order listed. Place the cover on the container. Turn on the blender and process by pressing the pulse button, while on the lowest blade-speed setting, until the ingredients are mostly blended. Continue mixing without the pulse function by pressing the highest blade-speed setting button until the mixture is smooth (it may be necessary to turn off the blender periodically and stir the mixture with a spoon, working from the bottom up). Turn off the blender. Pour the smoothie into a glass and garnish with a Crisp Blueberry Wafer (page 198), if desired.

Carb-on Copy

You can enjoy a serving of this cherry and berry refresher and then guiltlessly duplicate the pleasure with another glassful.

1 SERVING

½ cup diet cherry soda
2 tablespoons sugar-free blueberry syrup
6 tablespoons partially frozen raspberries
2 tablespoons partially frozen blueberries
1 scoop vanilla-flavored Atkins (or favorite low-carb) shake mix
½ to 1 teaspoon sugar-free raspberry Jell-O powder

Place all the ingredients in a blender container in the order listed. Place the cover on the container. Turn on the blender and process by pressing the pulse button, while on the lowest blade-speed setting, until the ingredients are mostly blended. Continue mixing without the pulse function by pressing the highest blade-speed setting button until the mixture is smooth (it may be necessary to turn off the blender periodically and stir the mixture with a spoon, working from the bottom up). Turn off the blender. Pour the smoothie into a glass and garnish with a Crisp Strawberry Wafer (page 198), if desired.

Carb Talk

This week's puzzler is to figure out why raspberries and strawberries, when combined with other low-carb ingredients, make such an incredibly tasty smoothie. Place these magical ingredients in a blender, identify the High button, and then tap it, brother.

1 SERVING

1/2 cup French vanilla-flavored AdvantEdge Carb
   Control (or favorite low-carb) ready-to-drink shake
2 tablespoons sugar-free mango syrup
1/4 cup low-carb raspberry yogurt
6 tablespoons partially frozen raspberries
1/4 cup partially frozen diced strawberries
1/2 teaspoon sugar-free raspberry Jell-O powder

Place all the ingredients in a blender container in the order listed. Place the cover on the container. Turn on the blender and process by pressing the pulse button, while on the lowest blade-speed setting, until the ingredients are mostly blended. Continue mixing without the pulse function by pressing the highest blade-speed setting button until the mixture is smooth (it may be necessary to turn off the blender periodically and stir the mixture with a spoon, working from the bottom up). Turn off the blender. Pour the smoothie into a glass and garnish with a Pecan Cookie on a Skewer (page 203), if desired.

Carb Your Appetite

This raspberry and apricot smoothie is the perfect elixir when you're feeling the urge to enjoy a drink that's rich and filling.

1 SERVING

½ cup French vanilla–flavored AdvantEdge Carb
    Control (or favorite low-carb) ready-to-drink shake
2 tablespoons sugar-free raspberry syrup
2 tablespoons heavy cream (or Carb Countdown
    dairy beverage)
6 tablespoons partially frozen raspberries
2 tablespoons partially frozen diced apricots
½ teaspoon sugar-free raspberry Jell-O powder

Place all the ingredients in a blender container in the order listed. Place the cover on the container. Turn on the blender and process by pressing the pulse button, while on the lowest blade-speed setting, until the ingredients are mostly blended. Continue mixing without the pulse function by pressing the highest blade-speed setting button until the mixture is smooth (it may be necessary to turn off the blender periodically and stir the mixture with a spoon, working from the bottom up). Turn off the blender. Pour the smoothie into a glass and garnish with Berries on a Skewer (page 189), if desired.

Eerie Cherry Berry

⟨⎯⎯⎯⎯⎯⎯⟩

This raspberry, cherry, and strawberry tropical smoothie is certain to send a chill up your spine.

1 SERVING

6 tablespoons Carb Countdown (or favorite low-carb) dairy beverage

3 tablespoons sugar-free cherry syrup

¼ cup partially frozen raspberries

¼ cup partially frozen diced strawberries

2 tablespoons ⅓-less-fat cream cheese

½ cup crushed frozen Minute Maid Light mango tropical (or favorite low-carb) fruit drink cubes

1 teaspoon sugar-free cherry Jell-O powder

Place all the ingredients in a blender container in the order listed. Place the cover on the container. Turn on the blender and process by pressing the pulse button, while on the lowest blade-speed setting, until the ingredients are mostly blended. Continue mixing without the pulse function by pressing the highest blade-speed setting button until the mixture is smooth (it may be necessary to turn off the blender periodically and stir the mixture with a spoon, working from the bottom up). Turn off the blender. Pour the smoothie into a glass and garnish with a Crisp Strawberry Wafer (page 198), if desired.

House of Carbs

Avoid a collapse from low-carb boredom by indulging in this amazingly flavorful ultra low-carb strawberry and kiwi treat.

1 SERVING

4 to 6 tablespoons strawberry kiwi (or favorite flavor) Crystal Light soft drink

2 tablespoons sugar-free strawberry syrup

6 tablespoons partially frozen diced strawberries

2 tablespoons partially frozen diced kiwi

1 scoop Zone Perfect (or favorite low-carb) protein powder

$\frac{1}{2}$ teaspoon sugar-free cherry Jell-O powder

$\frac{1}{4}$ teaspoon ground cinnamon

$\frac{1}{8}$ teaspoon ground ginger

Place all the ingredients in a blender container in the order listed. Place the cover on the container. Turn on the blender and process by pressing the pulse button, while on the lowest blade-speed setting, until the ingredients are mostly blended. Continue mixing without the pulse function by pressing the highest blade-speed setting button until the mixture is smooth (it may be necessary to turn off the blender periodically and stir the mixture with a spoon, working from the bottom up). Turn off the blender. Pour the smoothie into a glass and garnish with a Peanut Butter Cookie on a Skewer (page 201), if desired.

Huckleberry Thin

If you're looking for adventure, rev up a glassful of this delicious raspberry and blueberry blend. It's low-carb, but sweet and flavorful. Who said never the Twain shall meet?

1 SERVING

8 to 10 tablespoons raspberry ice (or favorite flavor) Crystal Light soft drink

2 tablespoons sugar-free blueberry syrup

6 tablespoons partially frozen raspberries

2 tablespoons partially frozen blueberries

1 to 2 scoops vanilla-flavored KĒTO (or favorite low-carb) shake

½ to 1 teaspoon sugar-free raspberry Jell-O powder

Place all the ingredients in a blender container in the order listed. Place the cover on the container. Turn on the blender and process by pressing the pulse button, while on the lowest blade-speed setting, until the ingredients are mostly blended. Continue mixing without the pulse function by pressing the highest blade-speed setting button until the mixture is smooth (it may be necessary to turn off the blender periodically and stir the mixture with a spoon, working from the bottom up). Turn off the blender. Pour the smoothie into a glass and garnish with a Crisp Blueberry Wafer (page 198), if desired.

I Left My Carbs in San Francisco

High on a chill, this raspberry and blueberry smoothie calls for you to indulge in its delightful combination of flavors.

1 SERVING

6 tablespoons diet cherry soda
2 tablespoons sugar-free raspberry syrup
6 tablespoons partially frozen raspberries
2 tablespoons partially frozen blueberries
½ cup crushed frozen Minute Maid Light mango tropical (or favorite low-carb) fruit drink cubes
½ to 1 teaspoon sugar-free raspberry Jell-O powder

Place all the ingredients in a blender container in the order listed. Place the cover on the container. Turn on the blender and process by pressing the pulse button, while on the lowest blade-speed setting, until the ingredients are mostly blended. Continue mixing without the pulse function by pressing the highest blade-speed setting button until the mixture is smooth (it may be necessary to turn off the blender periodically and stir the mixture with a spoon, working from the bottom up). Turn off the blender. Pour the smoothie into a glass and garnish with a Chocolate Chip Meringue on a Skewer (page 190), if desired.

Man! I Peel Like a Woman

Being on a low-carb diet doesn't mean you're immune to having a little fun, so let it all hang out with this raspberry and orange smoothie.

1 SERVING

4 to 6 tablespoons diet orange soda
2 tablespoons sugar-free cherry syrup
6 tablespoons partially frozen raspberries
2 tablespoons partially frozen diced orange
1 scoop Zone Perfect (or favorite low-carb)
    protein powder
½ to 1 teaspoon sugar-free orange Jell-O powder

Place all the ingredients in a blender container in the order listed. Place the cover on the container. Turn on the blender and process by pressing the pulse button, while on the lowest blade-speed setting, until the ingredients are mostly blended. Continue mixing without the pulse function by pressing the highest blade-speed setting button until the mixture is smooth (it may be necessary to turn off the blender periodically and stir the mixture with a spoon, working from the bottom up). Turn off the blender. Pour the smoothie into a glass and garnish the rim with an Orange Wheel (page 200), if desired.

Peter, Paul, and Berry

"Don't Think Twice, It's All Right" to indulge in this folksy strawberry smoothie with almond overtones.

1 SERVING

6 tablespoons Carb Countdown (or favorite low-carb) dairy beverage
2 tablespoons sugar-free strawberry syrup
2 tablespoons sugar-free almond syrup
½ cup partially frozen diced strawberries

Place all the ingredients in a blender container in the order listed. Place the cover on the container. Turn on the blender and process by pressing the pulse button, while on the lowest blade-speed setting, until the ingredients are mostly blended. Continue mixing without the pulse function by pressing the highest blade-speed setting button until the mixture is smooth (it may be necessary to turn off the blender periodically and stir the mixture with a spoon, working from the bottom up). Turn off the blender. Pour the smoothie into a glass and garnish the rim with a Strawberry Fan (page 205), if desired.

Raspberry Carb Lite

This light-bodied raspberry refresher has a smooth mouthfeel and is even smoother going down. Bottoms up!

1 SERVING

4 to 6 tablespoons diet cherry soda

3 tablespoons sugar-free raspberry syrup

1/2 cup partially frozen raspberries

1 scoop Zone Perfect (or favorite low-carb)
   protein powder

1/2 teaspoon sugar-free cherry Jell-O powder

1/2 cup crushed frozen Old Orchard Lo Carb apple
   raspberry juice cocktail blend (or favorite low-carb
   juice) cubes

Place all the ingredients in a blender container in the order listed. Place the cover on the container. Turn on the blender and process by pressing the pulse button, while on the lowest blade-speed setting, until the ingredients are mostly blended. Continue mixing without the pulse function by pressing the highest blade-speed setting button until the mixture is smooth (it may be necessary to turn off the blender periodically and stir the mixture with a spoon, working from the bottom up). Turn off the blender. Pour the smoothie into a glass and garnish with an Apple Chip (page 187), if desired.

Raspberry Carb Shark

This intensely flavored smoothie is unbelievably a five-carb draw. Serve it to friends just
once, and you're always certain to have a full
house.

1 SERVING

½ cup Carb Countdown (or favorite low-carb)
    dairy beverage
2 tablespoons sugar-free raspberry syrup
½ cup partially frozen raspberries
½ cup crushed frozen Minute Maid Light raspberry
    passion (or favorite low-carb) fruit drink cubes
½ teaspoon sugar-free raspberry Jell-O powder

Place all the ingredients in a blender container in the
order listed. Place the cover on the container. Turn on
the blender and process by pressing the pulse button,
while on the lowest blade-speed setting, until the ingredients are mostly blended. Continue mixing without
the pulse function by pressing the highest blade-speed
setting button until the mixture is smooth (it may be
necessary to turn off the blender periodically and stir
the mixture with a spoon, working from the bottom
up). Turn off the blender. Pour the smoothie into a
glass and garnish with a Pecan Cookie on a Skewer
(page 203), if desired.

Raspberry Cyber Carbs

Get on the chat board and spread the word about this fantastic low-carb raspberry and strawberry smoothie.

1 SERVING

½ cup French vanilla–flavored AdvantEdge Carb Control (or favorite low-carb) ready-to-drink shake

2 tablespoons sugar-free raspberry syrup

2 tablespoons heavy cream (or Carb Countdown dairy beverage)

¼ cup partially frozen diced strawberries

¼ cup partially frozen raspberries

½ teaspoon sugar-free strawberry Jell-O powder

Place all the ingredients in a blender container in the order listed. Place the cover on the container. Turn on the blender and process by pressing the pulse button, while on the lowest blade-speed setting, until the ingredients are mostly blended. Continue mixing without the pulse function by pressing the highest blade-speed setting button until the mixture is smooth (it may be necessary to turn off the blender periodically and stir the mixture with a spoon, working from the bottom up). Turn off the blender. Pour the smoothie into a glass and garnish the rim with a Strawberry Fan (page 205), if desired.

Slim Dandy

When you're feeling like you're about to cave in to temptation, it's Slim Dandy to the rescue. This creamy raspberry and blackberry smoothie will satisfy both your hunger and your sweet tooth.

1 SERVING

¼ cup Carb Countdown (or favorite low-carb) dairy beverage
2 tablespoons diet cherry soda
2 tablespoons sugar-free cherry syrup
6 tablespoons partially frozen raspberries
2 tablespoons partially frozen blackberries
1 scoop vanilla-flavored KĒTO
    (or favorite low-carb) shake
½ teaspoon sugar-free cherry Jell-O powder

Place all the ingredients in a blender container in the order listed. Place the cover on the container. Turn on the blender and process by pressing the pulse button, while on the lowest blade-speed setting, until the ingredients are mostly blended. Continue mixing without the pulse function by pressing the highest blade-speed setting button until the mixture is smooth (it may be necessary to turn off the blender periodically and stir the mixture with a spoon, working from the bottom up). Turn off the blender. Pour the smoothie into a glass and garnish with a Peanut Butter Cookie on a Skewer (page 201), if desired.

Strawberry Blizzard of Oz

With just a little heart, courage, and a brain, you can start a blizzard in your kitchen. Just click your shoes, add strawberries, heavy cream, and cherry soda to your blender, and follow the mellow drink road.

1 SERVING

¼ cup diet cherry soda
2 tablespoons sugar-free cherry syrup
2 tablespoons heavy cream (or Carb Countdown dairy beverage)
½ cup partially frozen diced strawberries
2 tablespoons ⅓-less-fat cream cheese
½ teaspoon sugar-free cherry Jell-O powder

Place all the ingredients in a blender container in the order listed. Place the cover on the container. Turn on the blender and process by pressing the pulse button, while on the lowest blade-speed setting, until the ingredients are mostly blended. Continue mixing without the pulse function by pressing the highest blade-speed setting button until the mixture is smooth (it may be necessary to turn off the blender periodically and stir the mixture with a spoon, working from the bottom up). Turn off the blender. Pour the smoothie into a glass and garnish the rim with a Strawberry Fan (page 205), if desired.

Strawberry Scorn on the Carb

You don't have to be from Iowa to enjoy this all-American strawberry and banana heart-land favorite.

1 SERVING

½ cup Carb Countdown (or favorite low-carb) dairy beverage
3 tablespoons sugar-free banana syrup
½ cup partially frozen diced strawberries
1 scoop vanilla-flavored Atkins (or favorite low-carb) shake mix
1 teaspoon sugar-free strawberry-banana Jell-O powder

Place all the ingredients in a blender container in the order listed. Place the cover on the container. Turn on the blender and process by pressing the pulse button, while on the lowest blade-speed setting, until the ingredients are mostly blended. Continue mixing without the pulse function by pressing the highest blade-speed setting button until the mixture is smooth (it may be necessary to turn off the blender periodically and stir the mixture with a spoon, working from the bottom up). Turn off the blender. Pour the smoothie into a glass and garnish with a Peanut Butter Cookie on a Skewer (page 201), if desired.

Strawberry Slim Dunk

You'll be amazed that this delectable smoothie is an official NBA (Naughty but Allowable) low-carb beverage.

1 SERVING

6 tablespoons strawberry kiwi
    (or favorite flavor) Crystal Light soft drink
2 tablespoons sugar-free strawberry syrup
2 tablespoons heavy cream
    (or Carb Countdown dairy beverage)
½ cup partially frozen diced strawberries
1 scoop vanilla-flavored Atkins
    (or favorite low-carb) shake mix
½ tablespoon KĒTO (or favorite low-carb)
    banana instant pudding powder
½ teaspoon sugar-free strawberry Jell-O powder
    (optional)

Place all the ingredients in a blender container in the order listed. Place the cover on the container. Turn on the blender and process by pressing the pulse button, while on the lowest blade-speed setting, until the ingredients are mostly blended. Continue mixing without the pulse function by pressing the highest blade-speed setting button until the mixture is smooth (it may be necessary to turn off the blender periodically and stir the mixture with a spoon, working from the bottom up). Turn off the blender. Pour the smoothie into a glass and garnish with a Crisp Strawberry Wafer (page 198), if desired.

Thin and Tonic

The next time you reach for this refreshing strawberry smoothie, think of it as a low-carb cocktail.

1 SERVING

6 tablespoons strawberry kiwi (or favorite flavor)
    Crystal Light soft drink
2 tablespoons sugar-free strawberry syrup
2 tablespoons heavy cream (or Carb Countdown
    dairy beverage)
½ cup partially frozen diced strawberries
1 scoop vanilla-flavored KĒTO
    (or favorite low-carb) shake
¼ to ½ teaspoon ground cinnamon, or to taste

Place all the ingredients in a blender container in the order listed. Place the cover on the container. Turn on the blender and process by pressing the pulse button, while on the lowest blade-speed setting, until the ingredients are mostly blended. Continue mixing without the pulse function by pressing the highest blade-speed setting button until the mixture is smooth (it may be necessary to turn off the blender periodically and stir the mixture with a spoon, working from the bottom up). Turn off the blender. Pour the smoothie into a glass and garnish with a Chocolate Chip Meringue on a Skewer (page 190), if desired.

War of the Whirls

No science fiction here. This extraordinary tropical smoothie actually has only 5 carbs.

1 SERVING

½ cup French vanilla-flavored AdvantEdge
   Carb Control (or favorite low-carb)
   ready-to-drink shake
2 tablespoons sugar-free mango syrup
½ cup partially frozen raspberries
¼ cup partially frozen diced strawberries
1 scoop Zone Perfect (or favorite low-carb)
   protein powder
½ teaspoon sugar-free lime Jell-O powder

Place all the ingredients in a blender container in the order listed. Place the cover on the container. Turn on the blender and process by pressing the pulse button, while on the lowest blade-speed setting, until the ingredients are mostly blended. Continue mixing without the pulse function by pressing the highest blade-speed setting button until the mixture is smooth (it may be necessary to turn off the blender periodically and stir the mixture with a spoon, working from the bottom up). Turn off the blender. Pour the smoothie into a glass and garnish the rim with an Orange Wheel (page 200), if desired.

Simple Pleasures

———

LOW-CARB SMOOTHIES

These smoothies
have *10* grams
of carbohydrates
or less.

Ain't No Big Peel

Whoever said it was difficult to stay on the low-carb regimen hadn't tasted an orange and strawberry smoothie gussied up with low-carb ice cream. I think I like this diet!

1 SERVING

6 to 8 tablespoons diet orange soda
2 tablespoons sugar-free strawberry syrup
$\frac{1}{4}$ cup partially frozen diced strawberries
$\frac{1}{4}$ cup partially frozen diced orange
$\frac{1}{4}$ cup low-carb strawberry ice cream
$\frac{1}{2}$ to 1 teaspoon sugar-free strawberry Jell-O powder

Place all the ingredients in a blender container in the order listed. Place the cover on the container. Turn on the blender and process by pressing the pulse button, while on the lowest blade-speed setting, until the ingredients are mostly blended. Continue mixing without the pulse function by pressing the highest blade-speed setting button until the mixture is smooth (it may be necessary to turn off the blender periodically and stir the mixture with a spoon, working from the bottom up). Turn off the blender. Pour the smoothie into a glass and garnish the rim with an Orange Wheel (page 200), if desired.

Berries in the Zone

Follow the guidelines for drinking this sensational blueberry and raspberry smoothie and it will help you achieve and maintain your Zone-perfect weight.

1 SERVING

¼ cup strawberry kiwi (or favorite flavor)
   Crystal Light soft drink
3 tablespoons sugar-free raspberry syrup
½ cup low-carb strawberry yogurt
6 tablespoons partially frozen raspberries
2 tablespoons partially frozen blueberries
1 scoop Zone Perfect (or favorite low-carb)
   protein powder
½ teaspoon sugar-free strawberry Jell-O powder

Place all the ingredients in a blender container in the order listed. Place the cover on the container. Turn on the blender and process by pressing the pulse button, while on the lowest blade-speed setting, until the ingredients are mostly blended. Continue mixing without the pulse function by pressing the highest blade-speed setting button until the mixture is smooth (it may be necessary to turn off the blender periodically and stir the mixture with a spoon, working from the bottom up). Turn off the blender. Pour the smoothie into a glass and garnish with a Chocolate Chip Meringue on a Skewer (page 190), if desired.

Berry-atrics

This refreshing blueberry and strawberry smoothie will never be "weight-listed" because it's heavy on flavor and light in carbs and calories.

1 SERVING

6 tablespoons Carb Countdown (or favorite low-carb) dairy beverage
2 tablespoons sugar-free blueberry syrup
¼ cup partially frozen diced strawberries
¼ cup partially frozen blueberries
½ teaspoon sugar-free strawberry Jell-O powder

Place all the ingredients in a blender container in the order listed. Place the cover on the container. Turn on the blender and process by pressing the pulse button, while on the lowest blade-speed setting, until the ingredients are mostly blended. Continue mixing without the pulse function by pressing the highest blade-speed setting button until the mixture is smooth (it may be necessary to turn off the blender periodically and stir the mixture with a spoon, working from the bottom up). Turn off the blender. Pour the smoothie into a glass and garnish with a Crisp Strawberry Wafer (page 198), if desired.

A Berry Chocolate Smoothie

You'll be "berry" happy to know it isn't naughty to indulge in this low-carb, chocolate, raspberry, and strawberry smoothie.

1 SERVING

¼ cup Carb Countdown (or favorite low-carb) dairy beverage
2 tablespoons sugar-free chocolate syrup
½ cup low-carb raspberry yogurt
½ cup partially frozen diced strawberries
¼ cup partially frozen raspberries

Place all the ingredients in a blender container in the order listed. Place the cover on the container. Turn on the blender and process by pressing the pulse button, while on the lowest blade-speed setting, until the ingredients are mostly blended. Continue mixing without the pulse function by pressing the highest blade-speed setting button until the mixture is smooth (it may be necessary to turn off the blender periodically and stir the mixture with a spoon, working from the bottom up). Turn off the blender. Pour the smoothie into a glass and serve with a Chocolate-Covered Spoon (page 192), if desired.

Berry Had a Little Lamb

This fruit-filled masterpiece is so addictive, you'll soon find that everywhere the berries went, your limbs are sure to go.

1 SERVING

¼ cup diet cherry soda
3 tablespoons sugar-free almond syrup
½ cup low-carb raspberry yogurt
6 tablespoons partially frozen raspberries
2 tablespoons partially frozen blueberries
1 scoop Zone Perfect (or favorite low-carb) protein powder
½ teaspoon sugar-free raspberry Jell-O powder

Place all the ingredients in a blender container in the order listed. Place the cover on the container. Turn on the blender and process by pressing the pulse button, while on the lowest blade-speed setting, until the ingredients are mostly blended. Continue mixing without the pulse function by pressing the highest blade-speed setting button until the mixture is smooth (it may be necessary to turn off the blender periodically and stir the mixture with a spoon, working from the bottom up). Turn off the blender. Pour the smoothie into a glass and garnish with a Peanut Butter Cookie on a Skewer (page 201), if desired.

Blueberry Chill

On days when your willpower is weakening, you'll find a low-carb thrill with Blueberry Chill.

1 SERVING

$\frac{1}{4}$ cup Carb Countdown (or favorite low-carb) dairy beverage
3 tablespoons sugar-free blueberry syrup
$\frac{1}{4}$ cup partially frozen blueberries
$\frac{1}{4}$ cup partially frozen raspberries
$\frac{1}{4}$ cup low-carb strawberry ice cream

Place all the ingredients in a blender container in the order listed. Place the cover on the container. Turn on the blender and process by pressing the pulse button, while on the lowest blade-speed setting, until the ingredients are mostly blended. Continue mixing without the pulse function by pressing the highest blade-speed setting button until the mixture is smooth (it may be necessary to turn off the blender periodically and stir the mixture with a spoon, working from the bottom up). Turn off the blender. Pour the smoothie into a glass and garnish with a Pecan Cookie on a Skewer (page 203), if desired.

Chilling Me Softly with Oranges

Don't believe that citrus must always be off-limits for your diet. Even with juicy oranges, this amazingly flavorful refresher weighs in at less than 11 carbs.

1 SERVING

½ cup French vanilla-flavored AdvantEdge Carb
    Control (or favorite low-carb) ready-to-drink shake
2 tablespoons sugar-free cherry syrup
¼ cup low-carb raspberry yogurt
¼ cup partially frozen diced orange
¼ cup partially frozen raspberries
½ teaspoon sugar-free orange Jell-O powder

Place all the ingredients in a blender container in the order listed. Place the cover on the container. Turn on the blender and process by pressing the pulse button, while on the lowest blade-speed setting, until the ingredients are mostly blended. Continue mixing without the pulse function by pressing the highest blade-speed setting button until the mixture is smooth (it may be necessary to turn off the blender periodically and stir the mixture with a spoon, working from the bottom up). Turn off the blender. Pour the smoothie into a glass and garnish the rim with an Orange Wheel (page 200), if desired.

Hic-kiwi
Dic-kiwi Dock

You won't have to wait for the clock to strike one to enjoy this delightful kiwi and raspberry smoothie. It's so low in carbs, you can drink it any time of the day.

1 SERVING

$\frac{1}{4}$ cup strawberry kiwi (or favorite flavor) Crystal Light soft drink

2 tablespoons sugar-free raspberry syrup

2 tablespoons heavy cream (or Carb Countdown dairy beverage)

$\frac{1}{4}$ cup partially frozen raspberries

$\frac{1}{4}$ cup partially frozen diced kiwi

1 scoop Zone Perfect (or favorite low-carb) protein powder

1 teaspoon sugar-free raspberry Jell-O powder

Place all the ingredients in a blender container in the order listed. Place the cover on the container. Turn on the blender and process by pressing the pulse button, while on the lowest blade-speed setting, until the ingredients are mostly blended. Continue mixing without the pulse function by pressing the highest blade-speed setting button until the mixture is smooth (it may be necessary to turn off the blender periodically and stir the mixture with a spoon, working from the bottom up). Turn off the blender. Pour the smoothie into a glass and garnish with a Pear Chip (page 187), if desired.

Low-Carb Berry-go-round

This dizzying concoction of strawberries and blackberries puts a new spin on low-carb enjoyment.

1 SERVING

¼ cup raspberry ice (or favorite flavor) Crystal Light soft drink
2 tablespoons sugar-free cherry syrup
½ cup low-carb strawberry yogurt
¼ cup partially frozen blackberries
¼ cup partially frozen diced strawberries
½ teaspoon sugar-free strawberry Jell-O powder

Place all the ingredients in a blender container in the order listed. Place the cover on the container. Turn on the blender and process by pressing the pulse button, while on the lowest blade-speed setting, until the ingredients are mostly blended. Continue mixing without the pulse function by pressing the highest blade-speed setting button until the mixture is smooth (it may be necessary to turn off the blender periodically and stir the mixture with a spoon, working from the bottom up). Turn off the blender. Pour the smoothie into a glass and garnish with Berries on a Skewer (page 189), if desired.

A Low off Your Mind

There's no need to agonize over indulging in this creamy blueberry and raspberry smoothie. This stress-free glassful has less than 10 grams of carbs. Relax and enjoy!

1 SERVING

1/4 cup Carb Countdown (or favorite low-carb)
    dairy beverage
2 tablespoons sugar-free cherry syrup
1/2 cup low-carb raspberry yogurt
1/4 cup partially frozen blueberries
1/4 cup partially frozen raspberries
1/2 to 1 teaspoon sugar-free cherry Jell-O powder

Place all the ingredients in a blender container in the order listed. Place the cover on the container. Turn on the blender and process by pressing the pulse button, while on the lowest blade-speed setting, until the ingredients are mostly blended. Continue mixing without the pulse function by pressing the highest blade-speed setting button until the mixture is smooth (it may be necessary to turn off the blender periodically and stir the mixture with a spoon, working from the bottom up). Turn off the blender. Pour the smoothie into a glass and garnish with a Crisp Blueberry Wafer (page 198), if desired.

Low vs. Weighed

It won't take the Supreme Court to declare this richly flavored strawberry and blueberry smoothie legal on a low-carb diet. It's your choice.

1 SERVING

½ cup French vanilla-flavored AdvantEdge
    Carb Control (or favorite low-carb)
    ready-to-drink shake
2 tablespoons sugar-free blueberry syrup
½ cup low-carb strawberry yogurt
¼ cup partially frozen diced strawberries
¼ cup partially frozen blueberries
½ teaspoon sugar-free strawberry Jell-O powder

Place all the ingredients in a blender container in the order listed. Place the cover on the container. Turn on the blender and process by pressing the pulse button, while on the lowest blade-speed setting, until the ingredients are mostly blended. Continue mixing without the pulse function by pressing the highest blade-speed setting button until the mixture is smooth (it may be necessary to turn off the blender periodically and stir the mixture with a spoon, working from the bottom up). Turn off the blender. Pour the smoothie into a glass and garnish with a Crisp Strawberry Wafer (page 198), if desired.

Peach Credit Carb

Enjoy this low-carb peach and raspberry smoothie delight now, and you won't have to pay later.

1 SERVING

1/4 cup Carb Countdown (or favorite low-carb) dairy beverage
2 tablespoons sugar-free peach syrup
1/2 cup peach low-carb yogurt
1/4 cup partially frozen diced peach
1/4 cup partially frozen raspberries
1 teaspoon sugar-free peach Jell-O powder

Place all the ingredients in a blender container in the order listed. Place the cover on the container. Turn on the blender and process by pressing the pulse button, while on the lowest blade-speed setting, until the ingredients are mostly blended. Continue mixing without the pulse function by pressing the highest blade-speed setting button until the mixture is smooth (it may be necessary to turn off the blender periodically and stir the mixture with a spoon, working from the bottom up). Turn off the blender. Pour the smoothie into a glass and garnish with a Pecan Cookie on a Skewer (page 203), if desired.

Peach NASCARB

Being on a low-carb diet doesn't have to be a "drag." Enjoy this intensely flavored smoothie and discover that the race does go to the slimmest.

1 SERVING

4 to 6 tablespoons French vanilla–flavored
  AdvantEdge Carb Control (or favorite low-carb)
  ready-to-drink shake
2 tablespoons sugar-free peach syrup
½ cup low-carb peach yogurt
¼ cup partially frozen diced peach
¼ cup partially frozen raspberries
½ to 1 teaspoon sugar-free raspberry Jell-O powder

Place all the ingredients in a blender container in the order listed. Place the cover on the container. Turn on the blender and process by pressing the pulse button, while on the lowest blade-speed setting, until the ingredients are mostly blended. Continue mixing without the pulse function by pressing the highest blade-speed setting button until the mixture is smooth (it may be necessary to turn off the blender periodically and stir the mixture with a spoon, working from the bottom up). Turn off the blender. Pour the smoothie into a glass and garnish the rim with an Orange Wheel (page 200), if desired.

Peach Rent-a-Carb

Drink as much of this rich and creamy blend as you like—it never Hertz.

1 SERVING

¼ cup Carb Countdown (or favorite low-carb) dairy beverage

3 tablespoons sugar-free peach syrup

½ cup low-carb raspberry yogurt

6 tablespoons partially frozen raspberries

2 tablespoons partially frozen diced peach

1 scoop Zone Perfect (or favorite low-carb) protein powder

½ to 1 teaspoon sugar-free peach Jell-O powder

Place all the ingredients in a blender container in the order listed. Place the cover on the container. Turn on the blender and process by pressing the pulse button, while on the lowest blade-speed setting, until the ingredients are mostly blended. Continue mixing without the pulse function by pressing the highest blade-speed setting button until the mixture is smooth (it may be necessary to turn off the blender periodically and stir the mixture with a spoon, working from the bottom up). Turn off the blender. Pour the smoothie into a glass and garnish with Berries on a Skewer (page 189), if desired.

Pick a Carb, Any Carb

Your friends will think you're a magician when you offer them this amazing diet-friendly raspberry sensation. It disappears as soon as it's poured.

1 SERVING

- 4 to 6 tablespoons strawberry kiwi (or favorite flavor) Crystal Light soft drink
- 2 tablespoons sugar-free raspberry syrup
- ½ cup low-carb raspberry yogurt
- ½ cup partially frozen raspberries
- 1 scoop vanilla-flavored Atkins (or favorite low-carb) shake mix
- ½ teaspoon sugar-free raspberry Jell-O powder

Place all the ingredients in a blender container in the order listed. Place the cover on the container. Turn on the blender and process by pressing the pulse button, while on the lowest blade-speed setting, until the ingredients are mostly blended. Continue mixing without the pulse function by pressing the highest blade-speed setting button until the mixture is smooth (it may be necessary to turn off the blender periodically and stir the mixture with a spoon, working from the bottom up). Turn off the blender. Pour the smoothie into a glass and garnish with a Crisp Blueberry Wafer (page 198), if desired.

Raspberry Tornado

Caution! Severe "whether" warning. Should you have a high-carb, high-calorie shake or this carb-friendly version that tastes just as good?

1 SERVING

$\frac{1}{2}$ cup Minute Maid Light mango tropical (or favorite low-carb) fruit drink

2 tablespoons sugar-free coconut syrup

$\frac{1}{2}$ cup partially frozen raspberries

$\frac{1}{4}$ cup low-carb vanilla ice cream

1 scoop vanilla-flavored Atkins (or favorite low-carb) shake mix

Place all the ingredients in a blender container in the order listed. Place the cover on the container. Turn on the blender and process by pressing the pulse button, while on the lowest blade-speed setting, until the ingredients are mostly blended. Continue mixing without the pulse function by pressing the highest blade-speed setting button until the mixture is smooth (it may be necessary to turn off the blender periodically and stir the mixture with a spoon, working from the bottom up). Turn off the blender. Pour the smoothie into a glass and garnish the rim with an Orange Wheel (page 200), if desired.

Return to Slender

Put your own stamp on a diet that works. Start with this low-carb strawberry and almond smoothie. It really delivers.

1 SERVING

4 to 6 tablespoons strawberry kiwi (or favorite flavor)
    Crystal Light soft drink
2 tablespoons sugar-free almond syrup
$\frac{1}{2}$ cup low-carb strawberry yogurt
6 tablespoons partially frozen diced strawberries
1 scoop Zone Perfect (or favorite low-carb)
    protein powder
$\frac{1}{2}$ teaspoon sugar-free strawberry Jell-O powder

Place all the ingredients in a blender container in the order listed. Place the cover on the container. Turn on the blender and process by pressing the pulse button, while on the lowest blade-speed setting, until the ingredients are mostly blended. Continue mixing without the pulse function by pressing the highest blade-speed setting button until the mixture is smooth (it may be necessary to turn off the blender periodically and stir the mixture with a spoon, working from the bottom up). Turn off the blender. Pour the smoothie into a glass and garnish the rim with a Strawberry Fan (page 205), if desired.

Rin Thin-Thin

Stay doggedly committed to your low-carb lifestyle without giving up on taste by sampling this richly satisfying treat.

1 SERVING

½ cup Carb Countdown (or favorite low-carb) dairy beverage
2 to 3 tablespoons sugar-free mango syrup
¼ cup partially frozen raspberries
2 tablespoons partially frozen diced apricot
½ cup crushed frozen Minute Maid Light mango tropical (or favorite low-carb) fruit drink cubes
½ to 1 teaspoon sugar-free raspberry Jell-O powder

Place all the ingredients in a blender container in the order listed. Place the cover on the container. Turn on the blender and process by pressing the pulse button, while on the lowest blade-speed setting, until the ingredients are mostly blended. Continue mixing without the pulse function by pressing the highest blade-speed setting button until the mixture is smooth (it may be necessary to turn off the blender periodically and stir the mixture with a spoon, working from the bottom up). Turn off the blender. Pour the smoothie into a glass and garnish with a Peanut Butter Cookie on a Skewer (page 201), if desired.

South Peach to Diet For

Just what the doctor ordered. This wonderful peach and strawberry blend will be a best seller in any low-carb household.

1 SERVING

½ cup French vanilla-flavored AdvantEdge
   Carb Control (or favorite low-carb)
   ready-to-drink shake
2 tablespoons sugar-free peach syrup
½ cup low-carb peach yogurt
6 tablespoons partially frozen diced strawberries
2 tablespoons partially frozen diced peach
1 teaspoon sugar-free peach Jell-O powder

Place all the ingredients in a blender container in the order listed. Place the cover on the container. Turn on the blender and process by pressing the pulse button, while on the lowest blade-speed setting, until the ingredients are mostly blended. Continue mixing without the pulse function by pressing the highest blade-speed setting button until the mixture is smooth (it may be necessary to turn off the blender periodically and stir the mixture with a spoon, working from the bottom up). Turn off the blender. Pour the smoothie into a glass and garnish with a Crisp Strawberry Wafer (page 198), if desired.

Sweet-Carb Named Desire

Get on track with this blueberry and raspberry pleaser. At less than 9 carbs, it's the exact fare you'll need for your transfer to a serious low-carb plan.

1 SERVING

4 to 6 tablespoons strawberry kiwi (or favorite flavor) Crystal Light soft drink

2 tablespoons sugar-free raspberry syrup

½ cup low-carb raspberry yogurt

¼ cup partially frozen blueberries

¼ cup partially frozen raspberries

1 scoop vanilla-flavored Atkins (or favorite low-carb) shake mix

½ teaspoon sugar-free raspberry Jell-O powder

Place all the ingredients in a blender container in the order listed. Place the cover on the container. Turn on the blender and process by pressing the pulse button, while on the lowest blade-speed setting, until the ingredients are mostly blended. Continue mixing without the pulse function by pressing the highest blade-speed setting button until the mixture is smooth (it may be necessary to turn off the blender periodically and stir the mixture with a spoon, working from the bottom up). Turn off the blender. Pour the smoothie into a glass and garnish with a Crisp Blueberry Wafer (page 198), if desired.

There's Something About Berry

If you're pining for the smoothies you used to enjoy before going on the low-carb diet, you'll be happy to know that this ideal strawberry smoothie can be made in a zip and will quickly fulfill your desires.

1 SERVING

4 to 6 tablespoons strawberry kiwi (or favorite flavor)
   Crystal Light soft drink
2 tablespoons sugar-free strawberry syrup
1/2 cup low-carb peach yogurt
1/2 cup partially frozen diced strawberries
1 scoop vanilla-flavored Atkins (or favorite low-carb)
   shake mix
1/2 to 1 tablespoon KĒTO (or favorite low-carb)
   French vanilla instant pudding powder

Place all the ingredients in a blender container in the order listed. Place the cover on the container. Turn on the blender and process by pressing the pulse button, while on the lowest blade-speed setting, until the ingredients are mostly blended. Continue mixing without the pulse function by pressing the highest blade-speed setting button until the mixture is smooth (it may be necessary to turn off the blender periodically and stir the mixture with a spoon, working from the bottom up). Turn off the blender. Pour the smoothie into a glass and garnish with Berries on a Skewer (page 189), if desired.

· 5 ·

Frosty and Fortified

Pumped-Up Smoothies for Your Health

Tell me what you eat,
I'll tell you who you are.

—Anthelme Brillat-Savarin

IN THE PAST DECADE, SMOOTHIES HAVE BECOME the "in" drink for people of all dietary persuasions except one—the low-carb diet. Here's the dilemma: Most fruit is high in carbohydrates, and as a result, people who follow a low-carb plan are encouraged to limit the amount of this important food category in their diet. But it is widely agreed that regular servings of fruit are important to maintain a healthy lifestyle. Medical experts have warned us to avoid falling into the trap of eliminating healthful foods, such as fruit, from our menu in the name of cutting back on carbs.

Low-Carb Smoothies to the rescue! A well-conceived low-carb smoothie can be your ticket to fulfilling the American Cancer Institute's recommendation that you include at least two to three servings of fruit in your daily diet. As you'll see throughout *Low-Carb Smoothies,* this can be accomplished by blending reasonable portions of relatively low-carb fruit with other well-chosen carb-friendly ingredients. What's more important, with a spoonful or two of a well-chosen additive, the health benefits and energy boost derived from these new age smoothies can be programmed still higher.

In this chapter you will be delighted to find more than forty low-carb recipes designed for the health-conscious smoothie lovers among us who want a little more bang for their buck in a smoothie in terms of its nutritional value. Two of my favorites are the flavorful refresher It's Not Easy Being Lean, made with tofu, raspberries, flaxseed oil, and protein powder, and the soy protein–enhanced Backstreet Soys, a richly flavored smoothie made with soy milk, raspberries, blueberries, and Zone Perfect protein powder. No matter which recipes become your favorites, you'll find that the health- and energy-enhancing ingredients in these fruity blends never detract from their basic appeal. They are truly a dieter's dream come true—rich in taste, even more nutritionally satisfying than a regular smoothie, and low enough in carbohydrates so you can indulge in them any time of the day. Come aboard and begin to experience the satisfaction of knowing that you're doing something good for yourself with every delicious sip.

Frosty and Fortified

ULTRA LOW-CARB SMOOTHIES

These smoothies
have *8* grams
of carbohydrates
or less.

All That Razz

This raspberry smoothie is popular in Chicago and throughout the world. It's a real killer!

1 SERVING

½ cup diet orange soda
2 tablespoons sugar-free blueberry syrup
6 tablespoons partially frozen raspberries
1 scoop vanilla-flavored Amplify by Release
    (or favorite low-carb) dietary supplement
1 teaspoon sugar-free raspberry Jell-O powder
    (optional)

Place all the ingredients in a blender container in the order listed. Place the cover on the container. Turn on the blender and process by pressing the pulse button, while on the lowest blade-speed setting, until the ingredients are mostly blended. Continue mixing without the pulse function by pressing the highest blade-speed setting button until the mixture is smooth (it may be necessary to turn off the blender periodically and stir the mixture with a spoon, working from the bottom up). Turn off the blender. Pour the smoothie into a glass and garnish the rim with an Orange Wheel (page 200), if desired.

The Apprentice's Raspberry Smoothie

You're mired!!—in high-carb smoothies. Show some leadership by suggesting this low-carb berry and tofu alternative to your family and friends. You'll no longer have to be concerned about life in the bored room.

1 SERVING

⅓ cup firm tofu
½ cup diet orange soda
3 tablespoons sugar-free blueberry syrup
¼ cup partially frozen raspberries
1 scoop vanilla-flavored Atkins (or favorite low-carb) shake mix
1 teaspoon sugar-free raspberry Jell-O powder

Place the tofu in a blender container. Place the cover on the container. Turn on the blender and purée the tofu by pressing the lowest blade-speed setting button. Add the remaining ingredients in the order listed, and at the same blade-speed setting process by pressing the pulse button until the ingredients are mostly blended. Continue mixing without the pulse function by pressing the highest blade-speed setting button until the mixture is smooth (it may be necessary to turn off the blender periodically and stir the mixture with a spoon, working from the bottom up). Turn off the blender. Pour the smoothie into a glass and garnish with a Crisp Blueberry Wafer (page 198), if desired.

Backstreet Soys

"It's True!" This delicious smoothie made with soy milk, flaxseed oil, raspberries, and blueberries will be "the one" low-carb drink you'll make over and over again.

1 SERVING

½ cup sugar-free vanilla soy milk
3 tablespoons sugar-free cherry syrup
1 tablespoon flaxseed oil
¼ cup partially frozen raspberries
¼ cup partially frozen blueberries
1 scoop Zone Perfect (or favorite low-carb)
    protein powder
½ teaspoon sugar-free cherry Jell-O powder
    (optional)

Place all the ingredients in a blender container in the order listed. Place the cover on the container. Turn on the blender and process by pressing the pulse button, while on the lowest blade-speed setting, until the ingredients are mostly blended. Continue mixing without the pulse function by pressing the highest blade-speed setting button until the mixture is smooth (it may be necessary to turn off the blender periodically and stir the mixture with a spoon, working from the bottom up). Turn off the blender. Pour the smoothie into a glass and garnish with a Crisp Blueberry Wafer (page 198), if desired.

Berry Fuel-Efficient Carbs

The future is here now with this high-energy low-carb smoothie. You can say good-bye to the carb-guzzling store-bought variety.

1 SERVING

½ cup French vanilla–flavored AdvantEdge Carb Control (or favorite low-carb) ready-to-drink shake

2 tablespoons sugar-free blueberry syrup

¼ cup partially frozen blueberries

¼ cup partially frozen raspberries

1 scoop vanilla-flavored KĒTO (or favorite low-carb) shake

½ to 1 teaspoon sugar-free raspberry Jell-O powder (optional)

Place all the ingredients in a blender container in the order listed. Place the cover on the container. Turn on the blender and process by pressing the pulse button, while on the lowest blade-speed setting, until the ingredients are mostly blended. Continue mixing without the pulse function by pressing the highest blade-speed setting button until the mixture is smooth (it may be necessary to turn off the blender periodically and stir the mixture with a spoon, working from the bottom up). Turn off the blender. Pour the smoothie into a glass and garnish with a Crisp Blueberry Wafer (page 198), if desired.

Blue Lite Special

Attention, smoothie lovers! If you've been shopping around for an outstandingly rich blueberry and strawberry drink that's had its carbohydrates slashed, then rush over to the blender aisle in your kitchen. Such a deal!

1 SERVING

8 to 10 tablespoons diet orange soda

3 tablespoons sugar-free blueberry syrup

1/4 cup partially frozen diced strawberries

1/4 cup partially frozen blueberries

1 to 2 scoops vanilla-flavored KĒTO
     (or favorite low-carb) shake

1 teaspoon sugar-free strawberry Jell-O powder
     (optional)

1/2 teaspoon ground cinnamon (optional)

Place all the ingredients in a blender container in the order listed. Place the cover on the container. Turn on the blender and process by pressing the pulse button, while on the lowest blade-speed setting, until the ingredients are mostly blended. Continue mixing without the pulse function by pressing the highest blade-speed setting button until the mixture is smooth (it may be necessary to turn off the blender periodically and stir the mixture with a spoon, working from the bottom up). Turn off the blender. Pour the smoothie into a glass and garnish with a Crisp Strawberry Wafer (page 198), if desired.

A Carb for All Occasions

This berry and passion-fruit meal replacement is the hallmark of a successful low-carb lifestyle. One taste and you'll find that you've stopped greeting carbs forever.

1 SERVING

8 to 10 tablespoons Minute Maid Light raspberry passion (or favorite low-carb) fruit drink
2 tablespoons sugar-free blueberry syrup
6 tablespoons partially frozen raspberries
¼ cup partially frozen diced strawberries
2 scoops vanilla-flavored KĒTO (or favorite low-carb) shake
½ teaspoon sugar-free strawberry Jell-O powder (optional)

Place all the ingredients in a blender container in the order listed. Place the cover on the container. Turn on the blender and process by pressing the pulse button, while on the lowest blade-speed setting, until the ingredients are mostly blended. Continue mixing without the pulse function by pressing the highest blade-speed setting button until the mixture is smooth (it may be necessary to turn off the blender periodically and stir the mixture with a spoon, working from the bottom up). Turn off the blender. Pour the smoothie into a glass and garnish with a Crisp Strawberry Wafer (page 198), if desired.

The Carb-Sip Enterprise

Save some space after lunch for this coconut and strawberry power booster and you'll be beaming up and down the rest of the day.

1 SERVING

½ cup diet cherry soda
3 tablespoons sugar-free coconut syrup
½ cup partially frozen diced strawberries
1 scoop vanilla-flavored Amplify by Release
    (or favorite low-carb) dietary supplement
1 teaspoon sugar-free strawberry Jell-O powder

Place all the ingredients in a blender container in the order listed. Place the cover on the container. Turn on the blender and process by pressing the pulse button, while on the lowest blade-speed setting, until the ingredients are mostly blended. Continue mixing without the pulse function by pressing the highest blade-speed setting button until the mixture is smooth (it may be necessary to turn off the blender periodically and stir the mixture with a spoon, working from the bottom up). Turn off the blender. Pour the smoothie into a glass and garnish with a Peanut Butter Cookie on a Skewer (page 201), if desired.

Chicago Carbs

Forget the Billy Goat Curse. Enjoy a glass of this banana and berry winner in the friendly confines of your kitchen. On second thought, let's drink two!

1 SERVING

8 to 10 tablespoons diet cherry soda
2 tablespoons sugar-free banana syrup
½ cup partially frozen diced strawberries
¼ cup partially frozen raspberries
1 to 2 scoops vanilla-flavored KĒTO
   (or favorite low-carb) shake
1 teaspoon sugar-free strawberry-banana
   Jell-O powder (optional)

Place all the ingredients in a blender container in the order listed. Place the cover on the container. Turn on the blender and process by pressing the pulse button, while on the lowest blade-speed setting, until the ingredients are mostly blended. Continue mixing without the pulse function by pressing the highest blade-speed setting button until the mixture is smooth (it may be necessary to turn off the blender periodically and stir the mixture with a spoon, working from the bottom up). Turn off the blender. Pour the smoothie into a glass and garnish with Berries on a Skewer (page 189), if desired.

Curiouser and Curiouser Apricot Smoothie

Apricots in a low-carb smoothie? Yes, weighing in at an unbelievable 5.8 grams of carbohydrates, this delightful refresher gives you a taste of a previously forbidden fruit.

1 SERVING

6 to 8 tablespoons raspberry ice (or favorite flavor) Crystal Light soft drink
2 tablespoons sugar-free mango syrup
¼ cup partially frozen diced strawberries
¼ cup partially frozen diced apricot
1 to 2 scoops vanilla-flavored KĒTO (or favorite low-carb) shake
½ teaspoon sugar-free raspberry Jell-O powder (optional)

Place all the ingredients in a blender container in the order listed. Place the cover on the container. Turn on the blender and process by pressing the pulse button, while on the lowest blade-speed setting, until the ingredients are mostly blended. Continue mixing without the pulse function by pressing the highest blade-speed setting button until the mixture is smooth (it may be necessary to turn off the blender periodically and stir the mixture with a spoon, working from the bottom up). Turn off the blender. Pour the smoothie into a glass and garnish the rim with a Strawberry Fan (page 205), if desired.

Do Not Pass Low.
Do Not Collect 200 Carbs.

Don't roll the dice on high-carb snacks. Enjoying this energy-supplemented smoothie is better than owning the Electric Company, and what's more, you won't be leaving your diet to Chance.

1 SERVING

½ cup diet cherry soda
3 tablespoons sugar-free coconut syrup
6 tablespoons partially frozen diced strawberries
1 scoop vanilla-flavored Amplify by Release
   (or favorite low-carb) dietary supplement
1 teaspoon sugar-free strawberry Jell-O powder
   (optional)

Place all the ingredients in a blender container in the order listed. Place the cover on the container. Turn on the blender and process by pressing the pulse button, while on the lowest blade-speed setting, until the ingredients are mostly blended. Continue mixing without the pulse function by pressing the highest blade-speed setting button until the mixture is smooth (it may be necessary to turn off the blender periodically and stir the mixture with a spoon, working from the bottom up). Turn off the blender. Pour the smoothie into a glass and garnish with a Peanut Butter Cookie on a Skewer (page 201), if desired.

Flax or Better to Open

This healthful and delicious fruit and flaxseed oil combination is a hit in Vegas and elsewhere. You can bet on it.

1 SERVING

10 tablespoons diet cherry soda
3 tablespoons sugar-free pineapple syrup
1 tablespoon flaxseed oil
¼ cup partially frozen raspberries
2 tablespoons partially frozen blackberries
2 scoops vanilla-flavored KĒTO
   (or favorite low-carb) shake
1 teaspoon sugar-free raspberry Jell-O powder
   (optional)

Place all the ingredients in a blender container in the order listed. Place the cover on the container. Turn on the blender and process by pressing the pulse button, while on the lowest blade-speed setting, until the ingredients are mostly blended. Continue mixing without the pulse function by pressing the highest blade-speed setting button until the mixture is smooth (it may be necessary to turn off the blender periodically and stir the mixture with a spoon, working from the bottom up). Turn off the blender. Pour the smoothie into a glass and garnish with a Pear Chip (page 187), if desired.

Good Soy!

If your mission is to succeed on the low-carb diet, then treat yourself to this delicious smoothie made with soy milk, strawberries, and wheat bran.

1 SERVING

½ cup sugar-free vanilla soy milk
3 tablespoons sugar-free pineapple syrup
6 tablespoons partially frozen diced strawberries
1 scoop vanilla-flavored Atkins (or favorite low-carb) shake mix
1 tablespoon wheat bran
1 teaspoon sugar-free lime Jell-O powder (optional)

Place all the ingredients in a blender container in the order listed. Place the cover on the container. Turn on the blender and process by pressing the pulse button, while on the lowest blade-speed setting, until the ingredients are mostly blended. Continue mixing without the pulse function by pressing the highest blade-speed setting button until the mixture is smooth (it may be necessary to turn off the blender periodically and stir the mixture with a spoon, working from the bottom up). Turn off the blender. Pour the smoothie into a glass and garnish the rim with an Orange Wheel (page 200), if desired.

It's Not Easy Being Lean

Ever wonder why Kermit never gains weight? This raspberry smoothie made with tofu, flax-seed oil, raspberries, and protein powder makes weight loss entirely possible without aimlessly hopping around in search of a satisfying low-carb snack. Drink and enjoy!

1 SERVING

⅓ cup firm tofu

½ cup diet cherry soda

3 tablespoons sugar-free chocolate syrup

6 tablespoons partially frozen raspberries

1 scoop vanilla-flavored KĒTO (or favorite low-carb) shake

1 teaspoon sugar-free raspberry Jell-O powder

Place the tofu in a blender container. Place the cover on the container. Turn on the blender and purée the tofu by pressing the lowest blade-speed setting button. Add the remaining ingredients in the order listed, and at the same blade-speed setting process by pressing the pulse button until the ingredients are mostly blended. Continue mixing without the pulse function by pressing the highest blade-speed setting button until the mixture is smooth (it may be necessary to turn off the blender periodically and stir the mixture with a spoon, working from the bottom up). Turn off the blender. Pour the smoothie into a glass and garnish with 1 or 2 Chocolate-Dipped Marshmallows (page 194), if desired.

Jump for Soy

You'll be elated when you discover the low-carb count in this delicious raspberry smoothie made with soy milk and a healthy dose of flaxseed oil.

1 SERVING

½ cup sugar-free vanilla soy milk

3 tablespoons sugar-free blueberry syrup

1 tablespoon flaxseed oil

½ cup partially frozen raspberries

1 scoop Zone Perfect (or favorite low-carb) protein powder

1 teaspoon sugar-free raspberry Jell-O powder (optional)

Place all the ingredients in a blender container in the order listed. Place the cover on the container. Turn on the blender and process by pressing the pulse button, while on the lowest blade-speed setting, until the ingredients are mostly blended. Continue mixing without the pulse function by pressing the highest blade-speed setting button until the mixture is smooth (it may be necessary to turn off the blender periodically and stir the mixture with a spoon, working from the bottom up). Turn off the blender. Pour the smoothie into a glass and garnish with a Chocolate Chip Meringue on a Skewer (page 190), if desired.

The Last Straw

You've gained some weight and this time it's really the last straw! Not to worry. This strawberry- and apricot-laced smoothie sensation is so good that you are permitted to gulp without guilt.

1 SERVING

8 to 10 tablespoons diet orange soda
2 tablespoons sugar-free banana syrup
1/4 cup partially frozen diced strawberries
1/4 cup partially frozen diced apricot
1 to 2 scoops vanilla-flavored KĒTO
    (or favorite low-carb) shake
1 teaspoon sugar-free orange Jell-O powder
    (optional)

Place all the ingredients in a blender container in the order listed. Place the cover on the container. Turn on the blender and process by pressing the pulse button, while on the lowest blade-speed setting, until the ingredients are mostly blended. Continue mixing without the pulse function by pressing the highest blade-speed setting button until the mixture is smooth (it may be necessary to turn off the blender periodically and stir the mixture with a spoon, working from the bottom up). Turn off the blender. Pour the smoothie into a glass and garnish the rim with an Orange Wheel (page 200), if desired.

Lean for a Day

You may not win a washing machine, but this carb-friendly, chocolate-blueberry smoothie scores very high on the low-carb applause meter.

1 SERVING

½ cup Carb Countdown (or favorite low-carb)
   dairy beverage
2 tablespoons sugar-free chocolate syrup
2 tablespoons partially frozen blueberries
1 scoop vanilla-flavored Amplify by Release
   (or favorite low-carb) dietary supplement

Place all the ingredients in a blender container in the order listed. Place the cover on the container. Turn on the blender and process by pressing the pulse button, while on the lowest blade-speed setting, until the ingredients are mostly blended. Continue mixing without the pulse function by pressing the highest blade-speed setting button until the mixture is smooth (it may be necessary to turn off the blender periodically and stir the mixture with a spoon, working from the bottom up). Turn off the blender. Pour the smoothie into a glass and serve with a Chocolate-Covered Spoon (page 192), if desired.

Little Soy Blue

Start the morning with this blueberry and soy milk smoothie and you'll never be caught sleeping on the job.

1 SERVING

½ cup sugar-free vanilla soy milk
3 tablespoons sugar-free pineapple syrup
1 tablespoon flaxseed oil
6 tablespoons partially frozen blueberries
1 scoop Zone Perfect (or favorite low-carb)
    protein powder
1 teaspoon sugar-free cherry Jell-O powder (optional)

Place all the ingredients in a blender container in the order listed. Place the cover on the container. Turn on the blender and process by pressing the pulse button, while on the lowest blade-speed setting, until the ingredients are mostly blended. Continue mixing without the pulse function by pressing the highest blade-speed setting button until the mixture is smooth (it may be necessary to turn off the blender periodically and stir the mixture with a spoon, working from the bottom up). Turn off the blender. Pour the smoothie into a glass and garnish with Berries on a Skewer (page 189), if desired.

Low in the Dark

One taste of this brilliant raspberry and apricot smoothie made with tofu and protein powder and you'll feel an afterglow that lingers long after the last sip.

1 SERVING

⅓ cup firm tofu
6 tablespoons Minute Maid Light raspberry passion
    (or favorite low-carb) fruit drink
3 tablespoons sugar-free raspberry syrup
¼ cup partially frozen raspberries
¼ cup partially frozen diced apricot
1 scoop Zone Perfect (or favorite low-carb)
    protein powder
1 teaspoon sugar-free raspberry Jell-O powder
    (optional)

Place the tofu in a blender container. Place the cover on the container. Turn on the blender and purée the tofu by pressing the lowest blade-speed setting button. Add the remaining ingredients in the order listed, and at the same blade-speed setting process by pressing the pulse button until the ingredients are mostly blended. Continue mixing without the pulse function by pressing the highest blade-speed setting button until the mixture is smooth (it may be necessary to turn off the blender periodically and stir the mixture with a spoon, working from the bottom up). Turn off the blender. Pour the smoothie into a glass and garnish with an Apple Chip (page 187), if desired.

Peach Soys

Wouldn't it be nice to know why this smoothie is fun, fun, fun to drink? It's made with a blend of great-tasting and healthy soy milk and peach that makes it a natural for serving U.S.A.

1 SERVING

½ cup sugar-free vanilla soy milk
2 tablespoons sugar-free peach syrup
¼ cup partially frozen diced peach
1 scoop Zone Perfect (or favorite low-carb)
     protein powder
1 teaspoon sugar-free peach Jell-O powder (optional)

Place all the ingredients in a blender container in the order listed. Place the cover on the container. Turn on the blender and process by pressing the pulse button, while on the lowest blade-speed setting, until the ingredients are mostly blended. Continue mixing without the pulse function by pressing the highest blade-speed setting button until the mixture is smooth (it may be necessary to turn off the blender periodically and stir the mixture with a spoon, working from the bottom up). Turn off the blender. Pour the smoothie into a glass and garnish the rim with an Orange Wheel (page 200), if desired.

Rasp-ody in Blue

By George! This jazzy raspberry and blueberry smoothie is poised to become an undisputed low-carb American classic.

1 SERVING

8 to 10 tablespoons raspberry ice (or favorite flavor)
   Crystal Light soft drink
2 tablespoons sugar-free blueberry syrup
6 tablespoons partially frozen raspberries
2 tablespoons partially frozen blueberries
1 to 2 scoops vanilla-flavored KĒTO
   (or favorite low-carb) shake
½ to 1 teaspoon sugar-free raspberry Jell-O powder
   (optional)

Place all the ingredients in a blender container in the order listed. Place the cover on the container. Turn on the blender and process by pressing the pulse button, while on the lowest blade-speed setting, until the ingredients are mostly blended. Continue mixing without the pulse function by pressing the highest blade-speed setting button until the mixture is smooth (it may be necessary to turn off the blender periodically and stir the mixture with a spoon, working from the bottom up). Turn off the blender. Pour the smoothie into a glass and garnish with a Crisp Blueberry Wafer (page 198), if desired.

Skinny the Pooh

Since you can't have honey, say "hallo" to this surprisingly sweet raspberry and strawberry smoothie.

1 SERVING

$\frac{1}{2}$ cup sugar-free vanilla soy milk

2 tablespoons sugar-free raspberry syrup

$\frac{1}{4}$ cup partially frozen diced strawberries

$\frac{1}{4}$ cup partially frozen raspberries

1 scoop Zone Perfect (or favorite low-carb) protein powder

$\frac{1}{2}$ to 1 teaspoon sugar-free raspberry Jell-O powder (optional)

Place all the ingredients in a blender container in the order listed. Place the cover on the container. Turn on the blender and process by pressing the pulse button, while on the lowest blade-speed setting, until the ingredients are mostly blended. Continue mixing without the pulse function by pressing the highest blade-speed setting button until the mixture is smooth (it may be necessary to turn off the blender periodically and stir the mixture with a spoon, working from the bottom up). Turn off the blender. Pour the smoothie into a glass and garnish the rim with a Strawberry Fan (page 205), if desired.

Soy Meets Whirl

This low-carb smoothie, made with raspberries and soy milk, will be love at first glass.

1 SERVING

½ cup sugar-free vanilla soy milk
2 tablespoons diet cherry soda
3 tablespoons sugar-free mango syrup
½ cup partially frozen raspberries
2 scoops vanilla-flavored KĒTO
    (or favorite low-carb) shake
½ teaspoon sugar-free raspberry Jell-O powder
    (optional)

Place all the ingredients in a blender container in the order listed. Place the cover on the container. Turn on the blender and process by pressing the pulse button, while on the lowest blade-speed setting, until the ingredients are mostly blended. Continue mixing without the pulse function by pressing the highest blade-speed setting button until the mixture is smooth (it may be necessary to turn off the blender periodically and stir the mixture with a spoon, working from the bottom up). Turn off the blender. Pour the smoothie into a glass and garnish with a Pecan Cookie on a Skewer (page 203), if desired.

Strawberry MasterCarb

Strawberries: 3.6 carbs; KĒTO vanilla shake meal replacement: 0.5 carb; enjoying the intense flavors of kiwi, banana, and strawberry without gaining weight: priceless.

1 SERVING

8 to 10 tablespoons strawberry kiwi (or favorite flavor) Crystal Light soft drink

2 tablespoons sugar-free banana syrup

½ cup partially frozen diced strawberries

1 to 2 scoops vanilla-flavored KĒTO (or favorite low-carb) shake

½ to 1 teaspoon sugar-free strawberry Jell-O powder (optional)

Place all the ingredients in a blender container in the order listed. Place the cover on the container. Turn on the blender and process by pressing the pulse button, while on the lowest blade-speed setting, until the ingredients are mostly blended. Continue mixing without the pulse function by pressing the highest blade-speed setting button until the mixture is smooth (it may be necessary to turn off the blender periodically and stir the mixture with a spoon, working from the bottom up). Turn off the blender. Pour the smoothie into a glass and garnish with a Crisp Strawberry Wafer (page 198), if desired.

Strawberry Wheat 'n' Low

There's no substitute for real fiber in a healthy diet. Enjoy the taste and health-enhancing benefits of wheat bran in this banana and strawberry energy booster.

1 SERVING

$\frac{1}{2}$ cup Carb Countdown (or favorite low-carb) dairy beverage

3 tablespoons sugar-free banana syrup

1 tablespoon flaxseed oil

$\frac{1}{2}$ cup partially frozen diced strawberries

1 scoop Zone Perfect (or favorite low-carb) protein powder

1 tablespoon wheat bran

1 teaspoon sugar-free strawberry-banana Jell-O powder (optional)

Place all the ingredients in a blender container in the order listed. Place the cover on the container. Turn on the blender and process by pressing the pulse button, while on the lowest blade-speed setting, until the ingredients are mostly blended. Continue mixing without the pulse function by pressing the highest blade-speed setting button until the mixture is smooth (it may be necessary to turn off the blender periodically and stir the mixture with a spoon, working from the bottom up). Turn off the blender. Pour the smoothie into a glass and garnish with Berries on a Skewer (page 189), if desired.

Tofu or Not Tofu

That is the question. Whether it's nobler to just drink one glass of this flavorful low-carb smoothie or to consume two will be the happy dilemma of most people in your hamlet.

1 SERVING

⅓ cup firm tofu

½ cup diet orange soda

3 tablespoons sugar-free pineapple syrup

½ cup partially frozen diced strawberries

1 scoop Zone Perfect (or favorite low-carb) protein powder

½ teaspoon sugar-free strawberry Jell-O powder (optional)

Place the tofu in a blender container. Place the cover on the container. Turn on the blender and purée the tofu by pressing the lowest blade-speed setting button. Add the remaining ingredients in the order listed, and at the same blade-speed setting process by pressing the pulse button until the ingredients are mostly blended. Continue mixing without the pulse function by pressing the highest blade-speed setting button until the mixture is smooth (it may be necessary to turn off the blender periodically and stir the mixture with a spoon, working from the bottom up). Turn off the blender. Pour the smoothie into a glass and garnish with a Pecan Cookie on a Skewer (page 203), if desired.

Frosty and Fortified

LOW-CARB SMOOTHIES

These smoothies
have *12* grams
of carbohydrates
or less.

Apricot KĒTO the Kingdom

Anything you really need is yours in this cinnamon, apricot, and orange creation enhanced with a healthy dose of low-carb KĒTO protein.

1 SERVING

6 to 8 tablespoons diet orange soda

2 to 3 tablespoons sugar-free banana syrup

¼ cup partially frozen diced orange

¼ cup partially frozen diced apricot

1 to 2 scoops vanilla-flavored KĒTO
    (or favorite low-carb) shake

½ teaspoon ground cinnamon (optional)

Place all the ingredients in a blender container in the order listed. Place the cover on the container. Turn on the blender and process by pressing the pulse button, while on the lowest blade-speed setting, until the ingredients are mostly blended. Continue mixing without the pulse function by pressing the highest blade-speed setting button until the mixture is smooth (it may be necessary to turn off the blender periodically and stir the mixture with a spoon, working from the bottom up). Turn off the blender. Pour the smoothie into a glass and garnish the rim with an Orange Wheel (page 200), if desired.

Berry, Berry, Lite Contrary

Place all your smoothie ingredients in a row, add each one to a blender, and watch them grow into a bountiful strawberry and raspberry meal-in-a-glass.

1 SERVING

6 tablespoons diet cherry soda

2 tablespoons sugar-free cherry syrup

2 tablespoons $\frac{1}{3}$-less-fat cream cheese

$\frac{1}{4}$ cup partially frozen raspberries

$\frac{1}{4}$ cup partially frozen diced strawberries

1 scoop vanilla-flavored Amplify by Release
(or favorite low-carb) dietary supplement

$\frac{1}{2}$ teaspoon sugar-free raspberry Jell-O powder
(optional)

Place all the ingredients in a blender container in the order listed. Place the cover on the container. Turn on the blender and process by pressing the pulse button, while on the lowest blade-speed setting, until the ingredients are mostly blended. Continue mixing without the pulse function by pressing the highest blade-speed setting button until the mixture is smooth (it may be necessary to turn off the blender periodically and stir the mixture with a spoon, working from the bottom up). Turn off the blender. Pour the smoothie into a glass and garnish with a Pecan Cookie on a Skewer (page 203), if desired.

The Berry Thought of You

The subtle taste of kiwi enhances the strawberry essence of this unforgettable low-carb masterpiece.

1 SERVING

⅓ cup firm tofu

6 tablespoons French vanilla–flavored AdvantEdge Carb Control (or favorite low-carb) ready-to-drink shake

3 tablespoons sugar-free strawberry syrup

½ cup low-carb strawberry yogurt

¼ cup partially frozen diced strawberries

2 tablespoons partially frozen diced kiwi

½ teaspoon sugar-free strawberry Jell-O powder (optional)

Place the tofu in a blender container. Place the cover on the container. Turn on the blender and purée the tofu by pressing the lowest blade-speed setting button. Add the remaining ingredients in the order listed, and at the same blade-speed setting process by pressing the pulse button until the ingredients are mostly blended. Continue mixing without the pulse function by pressing the highest blade-speed setting button until the mixture is smooth (it may be necessary to turn off the blender periodically and stir the mixture with a spoon, working from the bottom up). Turn off the blender. Pour the smoothie into a glass and garnish with a Crisp Blueberry Wafer (page 198), if desired.

Carbaritaville

Don't be wastin' away in your kitchen search-in' for something good to drink. Rev up a glass of this frozen raspberry and blueberry concoction—it's a real beauty.

1 SERVING

½ cup Old Orchard Lo Carb apple raspberry juice cocktail blend (or favorite low-carb juice)

3 tablespoons sugar-free raspberry syrup

¼ cup partially frozen raspberries

¼ cup partially frozen blueberries

1 scoop vanilla-flavored Amplify by Release (or favorite low-carb) dietary supplement

½ teaspoon sugar-free raspberry Jell-O powder (optional)

Place all the ingredients in a blender container in the order listed. Place the cover on the container. Turn on the blender and process by pressing the pulse button, while on the lowest blade-speed setting, until the ingredients are mostly blended. Continue mixing without the pulse function by pressing the highest blade-speed setting button until the mixture is smooth (it may be necessary to turn off the blender periodically and stir the mixture with a spoon, working from the bottom up). Turn off the blender. Pour the smoothie into a glass and garnish with an Apple Chip (page 187), if desired.

Flax of Life

Forget the birds and the bees. It takes very little planning to reproduce the sensational flavors in this flax-enhanced raspberry and strawberry smoothie.

1 SERVING

1/4 cup French vanilla-flavored AdvantEdge Carb
   Control (or favorite low-carb) ready-to-drink shake
2 tablespoons sugar-free raspberry syrup
1/2 cup low-carb raspberry yogurt
1 tablespoon flaxseed oil
1/4 cup partially frozen raspberries
1/4 cup partially frozen diced strawberries
1/2 to 1 teaspoon sugar-free raspberry Jell-O powder
   (optional)

Place all the ingredients in a blender container in the order listed. Place the cover on the container. Turn on the blender and process by pressing the pulse button, while on the lowest blade-speed setting, until the ingredients are mostly blended. Continue mixing without the pulse function by pressing the highest blade-speed setting button until the mixture is smooth (it may be necessary to turn off the blender periodically and stir the mixture with a spoon, working from the bottom up). Turn off the blender. Pour the smoothie into a glass and garnish with a Peanut Butter Cookie on a Skewer (page 201), if desired.

I Peel Good Like I Knew I Would

The taste of this delicious low-carb orange and strawberry smoothie can be described in the immortal words of the Godfather of Soul—"Whoa-oa-oa-oa!"

1 SERVING

1/3 cup diet cherry soda
2 tablespoons sugar-free cherry syrup
1/4 cup partially frozen diced orange
1/4 cup partially frozen diced strawberries
1 scoop vanilla-flavored Amplify by Release
    (or favorite low-carb) dietary supplement
1 teaspoon sugar-free strawberry Jell-O powder
    (optional)

Place all the ingredients in a blender container in the order listed. Place the cover on the container. Turn on the blender and process by pressing the pulse button, while on the lowest blade-speed setting, until the ingredients are mostly blended. Continue mixing without the pulse function by pressing the highest blade-speed setting button until the mixture is smooth (it may be necessary to turn off the blender periodically and stir the mixture with a spoon, working from the bottom up). Turn off the blender. Pour the smoothie into a glass and garnish the rim with an Orange Wheel (page 200), if desired.

Low Is Me

When you're feeling a bit down, look to the brighter side by sampling this strawberry, pineapple, and orange protein-enhanced smoothie.

1 SERVING

½ cup diet orange soda
2 tablespoons sugar-free pineapple syrup
¼ cup partially frozen diced strawberries
¼ cup partially frozen diced orange
1 scoop vanilla-flavored Amplify by Release
(or favorite low-carb) dietary supplement
1 teaspoon sugar-free orange Jell-O powder
(optional)

Place all the ingredients in a blender container in the order listed. Place the cover on the container. Turn on the blender and process by pressing the pulse button, while on the lowest blade-speed setting, until the ingredients are mostly blended. Continue mixing without the pulse function by pressing the highest blade-speed setting button until the mixture is smooth (it may be necessary to turn off the blender periodically and stir the mixture with a spoon, working from the bottom up). Turn off the blender. Pour the smoothie into a glass and garnish with a Pear Chip (page 187), if desired.

No Shoes, No Shirt, Low Carb, No Problems

What better way to escape the daily routine than with a glass of this exotic apricot, strawberry, and pineapple smoothie meant to remind you of a tropical beach!

1 SERVING

¼ cup cottage cheese

½ cup French vanilla–flavored AdvantEdge Carb Control (or favorite low-carb) ready-to-drink shake

2 tablespoons sugar-free pineapple syrup

1 tablespoon flaxseed oil

6 tablespoons partially frozen diced strawberries

2 tablespoons partially frozen diced apricot

1 scoop Zone Perfect (or favorite low-carb) protein powder

1 teaspoon sugar-free orange Jell-O powder (optional)

Place the cottage cheese in a blender container. Place the cover on the container. Turn on the blender and purée the cottage cheese by pressing the lowest blade-speed setting button. Add the remaining ingredients in the order listed, and at the same blade-speed setting process by pressing the pulse button until the ingredients are mostly blended. Continue mixing without the pulse function by pressing the highest blade-speed setting button until the mixture is smooth (it may be necessary to turn off the blender periodically and stir the mixture with a spoon, working from the bottom up). Turn off the blender. Pour the smoothie into a glass and garnish the rim with an Orange Wheel (page 200), if desired.

Plum-dinger

This extraordinary protein-enhanced smoothie, made with cherry, plum, raspberry, and yogurt, is remarkable for its exceptional taste. Start the morning with a glassful and you won't be tempted to sneak a doughnut during your coffee break.

1 SERVING

½ cup French vanilla–flavored AdvantEdge Carb
    Control (or favorite low-carb) ready-to-drink shake
2 tablespoons sugar-free cherry syrup
½ cup low-carb peach or raspberry yogurt
¼ cup partially frozen diced plum
2 tablespoons partially frozen raspberries
1 scoop vanilla-flavored Amplify by Release
    (or favorite low-carb) dietary supplement
1 teaspoon sugar-free raspberry Jell-O powder
    (optional)

Place all the ingredients in a blender container in the order listed. Place the cover on the container. Turn on the blender and process by pressing the pulse button, while on the lowest blade-speed setting, until the ingredients are mostly blended. Continue mixing without the pulse function by pressing the highest blade-speed setting button until the mixture is smooth (it may be necessary to turn off the blender periodically and stir the mixture with a spoon, working from the bottom up). Turn off the blender. Pour the smoothie into a glass and garnish with Berries on a Skewer (page 189), if desired.

Putting the Carb Before the Porsche

You've got your priorities straight. Losing weight while enjoying this amplified kiwi and strawberry treat doesn't take a backseat to anything.

1 SERVING

½ cup strawberry kiwi (or favorite flavor) Crystal Light soft drink
2 tablespoons sugar-free strawberry syrup
½ cup low-carb strawberry yogurt
½ cup partially frozen diced strawberries
1 scoop vanilla-flavored Amplify by Release (or favorite low-carb) dietary supplement
½ teaspoon sugar-free strawberry-banana Jell-O powder (optional)

Place all thje ingredients in a blender container in the order listed. Place the cover on the container. Turn on the blender and process by pressing the pulse button, while on the lowest blade-speed setting, until the ingredients are mostly blended. Continue mixing without the pulse function by pressing the highest blade-speed setting button until the mixture is smooth (it may be necessary to turn off the blender periodically and stir the mixture with a spoon, working from the bottom up). Turn off the blender. Pour the smoothie into a glass and garnish with a Crisp Strawberry Wafer (page 198), if desired.

Raspberry Flax, Not Fiction

It's absolutely true that this soy, protein, and flax-fortified raspberry smoothie is high in energy but still under 10 carbs.

1 SERVING

½ cup sugar-free vanilla soy milk

3 tablespoons sugar-free raspberry syrup

1 tablespoon flaxseed oil

½ cup partially frozen raspberries

1 scoop vanilla-flavored Amplify by Release
   (or favorite low-carb) dietary supplement

½ teaspoon sugar-free raspberry Jell-O powder
   (optional)

Place all the ingredients in a blender container in the order listed. Place the cover on the container. Turn on the blender and process by pressing the pulse button, while on the lowest blade-speed setting, until the ingredients are mostly blended. Continue mixing without the pulse function by pressing the highest blade-speed setting button until the mixture is smooth (it may be necessary to turn off the blender periodically and stir the mixture with a spoon, working from the bottom up). Turn off the blender. Pour the smoothie into a glass and garnish with Berries on a Skewer (page 189), if desired.

Raspberry Orange Power Company

You'll experience a high-energy surge when you sample this amplified smoothie featuring oranges and raspberries.

1 SERVING

4 to 6 tablespoons raspberry ice (or favorite flavor) Crystal Light soft drink
2 tablespoons sugar-free cherry syrup
¼ cup partially frozen raspberries
¼ cup partially frozen diced orange
1 scoop vanilla-flavored Amplify by Release (or favorite low-carb) dietary supplement
½ to 1 teaspoon sugar-free orange Jell-O powder (optional)

Place all the ingredients in a blender container in the order listed. Place the cover on the container. Turn on the blender and process by pressing the pulse button, while on the lowest blade-speed setting, until the ingredients are mostly blended. Continue mixing without the pulse function by pressing the highest blade-speed setting button until the mixture is smooth (it may be necessary to turn off the blender periodically and stir the mixture with a spoon, working from the bottom up). Turn off the blender. Pour the smoothie into a glass and garnish with a Pecan Cookie on a Skewer (page 203), if desired.

Rind and Dined

You'll find this smoothie featuring juicy tangerines to be exciting and unusual. Add luscious strawberries and pump it up with protein powder—it's almost a meal but with a snack's worth of carbs.

1 SERVING

¼ cup strawberry tangerine (or favorite flavor) Crystal Light soft drink

2 tablespoons sugar-free strawberry syrup

½ cup low-carb strawberry yogurt

¼ cup partially frozen diced strawberries

2 tablespoons partially frozen diced tangerine

1 scoop vanilla-flavored Amplify by Release (or favorite low-carb) dietary supplement

½ teaspoon sugar-free orange Jell-O powder

Place all the ingredients in a blender container in the order listed. Place the cover on the container. Turn on the blender and process by pressing the pulse button, while on the lowest blade-speed setting, until the ingredients are mostly blended. Continue mixing without the pulse function by pressing the highest blade-speed setting button until the mixture is smooth (it may be necessary to turn off the blender periodically and stir the mixture with a spoon, working from the bottom up). Turn off the blender. Pour the smoothie into a glass and garnish with a Peanut Butter Cookie on a Skewer (page 201), if desired.

Romancing the Zone

You won't need to seek any greater treasure in your diet than this smoothie, featuring four fabulous fruit flavors combined with a fulfilling portion of carb-free Zone Perfect protein powder.

1 SERVING

⅓ cup firm tofu

6 tablespoons diet orange soda

3 tablespoons sugar-free banana syrup

¼ cup partially frozen raspberries

¼ cup partially frozen diced orange

1 scoop Zone Perfect (or favorite low-carb)
   protein powder

1 teaspoon sugar-free strawberry-banana
   Jell-O powder (optional)

Place the tofu in a blender container. Place the cover on the container. Turn on the blender and purée the tofu by pressing the lowest blade-speed setting button. Add the remaining ingredients in the order listed, and at the same blade-speed setting process by pressing the pulse button until the ingredients are mostly blended. Continue mixing without the pulse function by pressing the highest blade-speed setting button until the mixture is smooth (it may be necessary to turn off the blender periodically and stir the mixture with a spoon, working from the bottom up). Turn off the blender. Pour the smoothie into a glass and garnish the rim with an Orange Wheel (page 200), if desired.

Sipping the Lite Fantastic

Tap into the delicious flavors of coconut, peaches, cherries, and strawberries featured in this energy-supplemented smoothie and you'll be able to dance the night away.

1 SERVING

4 to 6 tablespoons diet cherry soda
2 tablespoons sugar-free coconut syrup
⅓ cup low-carb peach yogurt
¼ cup partially frozen diced strawberries
2 tablespoons partially frozen diced peach
1 scoop vanilla-flavored Amplify by Release
    (or favorite low-carb) dietary supplement
1 teaspoon sugar-free peach Jell-O powder
    (optional)

Place all the ingredients in a blender container in the order listed. Place the cover on the container. Turn on the blender and process by pressing the pulse button, while on the lowest blade-speed setting, until the ingredients are mostly blended. Continue mixing without the pulse function by pressing the highest blade-speed setting button until the mixture is smooth (it may be necessary to turn off the blender periodically and stir the mixture with a spoon, working from the bottom up). Turn off the blender. Pour the smoothie into a glass and garnish the rim with a Strawberry Fan (page 205), if desired.

Skinny Sipping

Take it off. Take it all off—pounds, that is—with this low-carb combination of raspberries and blueberries and a scoop of high-energy protein powder.

1 SERVING

$\frac{1}{2}$ cup Carb Countdown (or favorite low-carb) dairy beverage

2 tablespoons sugar-free chocolate syrup

$\frac{1}{4}$ cup partially frozen raspberries

$\frac{1}{4}$ cup partially frozen blueberries

1 scoop vanilla-flavored Amplify by Release (or favorite low-carb) dietary supplement

Place all the ingredients in a blender container in the order listed. Place the cover on the container. Turn on the blender and process by pressing the pulse button, while on the lowest blade-speed setting, until the ingredients are mostly blended. Continue mixing without the pulse function by pressing the highest blade-speed setting button until the mixture is smooth (it may be necessary to turn off the blender periodically and stir the mixture with a spoon, working from the bottom up). Turn off the blender. Pour the smoothie into a glass and garnish with a Chocolate Chip Meringue on a Skewer (page 190), if desired.

Slim the Lites

This blueberry and strawberry delicacy is the perfect snack and weighs in at under 7 carbs. Use it as a delicious hunger remedy between meals and you'll be delighted at how you tip the scale.

1 SERVING

⅓ cup firm tofu

½ cup French vanilla-flavored AdvantEdge Carb Control (or favorite low-carb) ready-to-drink shake

3 tablespoons sugar-free strawberry syrup

¼ cup partially frozen blueberries

¼ cup partially frozen diced strawberries

½ to 1 teaspoon sugar-free strawberry Jell-O powder (optional)

Place the tofu in a blender container. Place the cover on the container. Turn on the blender and purée the tofu by pressing the lowest blade-speed setting button. Add the remaining ingredients in the order listed, and at the same blade-speed setting process by pressing the pulse button until the ingredients are mostly blended. Continue mixing without the pulse function by pressing the highest blade-speed setting button until the mixture is smooth (it may be necessary to turn off the blender periodically and stir the mixture with a spoon, working from the bottom up). Turn off the blender. Pour the smoothie into a glass and garnish the rim with a Strawberry Fan (page 205), if desired.

A Soy Named Sue

Cash in on this mean raspberry and kiwi smoothie made with tofu and protein. It will help keep you strong and lean.

1 SERVING

⅓ cup firm tofu

½ cup strawberry kiwi (or favorite flavor) Crystal Light soft drink

3 tablespoons sugar-free raspberry syrup

6 tablespoons partially frozen raspberries

¼ cup partially frozen diced kiwi

1 scoop Zone Perfect (or favorite low-carb) protein powder

1 teaspoon sugar-free strawberry Jell-O powder (optional)

Place the tofu in a blender container. Place the cover on the container. Turn on the blender and purée the tofu by pressing the lowest blade-speed setting button. Add the remaining ingredients in the order listed, and at the same blade-speed setting process by pressing the pulse button until the ingredients are mostly blended. Continue mixing without the pulse function by pressing the highest blade-speed setting button until the mixture is smooth (it may be necessary to turn off the blender periodically and stir the mixture with a spoon, working from the bottom up). Turn off the blender. Pour the smoothie into a glass and garnish with Berries on a Skewer (page 189), if desired.

Strawberry No-Holds-Carbed

It may be difficult to restrain yourself from drinking another glassful of this strawberry smoothie because it's so tantalizingly delicious. Well, give in and enjoy—it's less than 10 carbs.

1 SERVING

1/2 cup sugar-free vanilla soy milk
3 tablespoons sugar-free raspberry syrup
1/2 cup partially frozen diced strawberries
1 scoop vanilla-flavored Amplify by Release
   (or favorite low-carb) dietary supplement
1 teaspoon sugar-free raspberry Jell-O powder
   (optional)

Place all the ingredients in a blender container in the order listed. Place the cover on the container. Turn on the blender and process by pressing the pulse button, while on the lowest blade-speed setting, until the ingredients are mostly blended. Continue mixing without the pulse function by pressing the highest blade-speed setting button until the mixture is smooth (it may be necessary to turn off the blender periodically and stir the mixture with a spoon, working from the bottom up). Turn off the blender. Pour the smoothie into a glass and garnish with a Crisp Strawberry Wafer (page 198), if desired.

Strawberry Peach Carb Blanche

You are under no restrictions when it comes to enjoying this carb-stingy raspberry, peach, and strawberry smoothie.

1 SERVING

8 to 10 tablespoons strawberry kiwi (or favorite flavor) Crystal Light soft drink
2 tablespoons sugar-free strawberry syrup
½ cup low-carb peach yogurt
¼ cup partially frozen diced strawberries
¼ cup partially frozen raspberries
2 scoops vanilla-flavored KĒTO (or favorite low-carb) shake
½ tablespoon KĒTO (or favorite low-carb) French vanilla instant pudding powder
½ teaspoon sugar-free raspberry Jell-O powder (optional)

Place all the ingredients in a blender container in the order listed. Place the cover on the container. Turn on the blender and process by pressing the pulse button, while on the lowest blade-speed setting, until the ingredients are mostly blended. Continue mixing without the pulse function by pressing the highest blade-speed setting button until the mixture is smooth (it may be necessary to turn off the blender periodically and stir the mixture with a spoon, working from the bottom up). Turn off the blender. Pour the smoothie into a glass and garnish with Berries on a Skewer (page 189), if desired.

The Whirl
According to Carb

Is this smoothie better than the book? Judge for yourself after tasting this intensely flavored strawberry creation fortified with protein.

1 SERVING

6 to 8 tablespoons strawberry kiwi (or favorite flavor)
    Crystal Light soft drink
2 tablespoons sugar-free strawberry syrup
$\frac{1}{2}$ cup partially frozen diced strawberries
1 scoop vanilla-flavored Amplify by Release
    (or favorite low-carb) dietary supplement
1 teaspoon sugar-free strawberry Jell-O powder
    (optional)

Place all the ingredients in a blender container in the order listed. Place the cover on the container. Turn on the blender and process by pressing the pulse button, while on the lowest blade-speed setting, until the ingredients are mostly blended. Continue mixing without the pulse function by pressing the highest blade-speed setting button until the mixture is smooth (it may be necessary to turn off the blender periodically and stir the mixture with a spoon, working from the bottom up). Turn off the blender. Pour the smoothie into a glass and garnish with a Crisp Strawberry Wafer (page 198), if desired.

Maintenance Low-Carb Smoothies

Now That You've Taken It Off, Keep It Off!

Never eat more than you can lift.

—Miss Piggy

IF YOU ARE A FORMER SMOOTHIE LOVER WHO has reached your target weight after religiously following a low-carb diet, then get ready to enjoy some heart-stopping glassfuls of low-carb ecstasy that will satisfy your urges but still help you keep the weight off. For those of you who simply need to maintain your current weight, not lose more, a slightly more liberal carb intake is acceptable, but without a good plan, this slight shift in diet strategy can quickly morph into a caloric disaster. To avoid this dilemma, the recipes in this chapter are characterized by a slightly more generous definition of "ultra low-carb" and "low-carb," but they still remain true to the low-carb philosophy.

With such a bounty of readily available snacks, sweets, and other high-carb enticements to lure us into submission, it's no wonder how quickly we can fall back into old eating habits. Who among us hasn't succumbed to tasting just one spoonful of a hot-fudge sundae, only to find that one spoonful led to another and then another, until the entire dessert was history. At last there is help to keep you from caving in to carb-laden temptations. As you browse through the recipes in this chapter, you'll see that by simply combining these fruits with a variety of well-chosen ingredients, such as low-carb ice cream, carb-light shakes, natural peanut butter, or sugar-free syrups, you can create an extraordinarily rich and creamy smoothie that will make you forget all things Krispy and Kreme-y.

Keep in mind that if you find the less drastically reduced carb count in this chapter's recipes too liberal, you can substitute lower-carb ingredients such as Crystal Light soft drinks in place of the low-carb dairy beverage or slightly reduce the amount of one or more ingredients, such as the low-carb ice cream. These steps will not only further restrict the carbs, they will also reduce the number of calories consumed.

Get ready to drool over forty-one mouthwatering smoothies featured in this chapter of endless low-carb pleasures and satisfaction. Here you'll find Just Say Low!, a kiwi and blueberry smoothie made with raspberry sorbet, as well as Uptown Whirl, a strawberry ice cream and blueberry smoothie featuring peanut butter. Go ahead and splurge ever so slightly on these low-carb delights and you won't be tempted by truly sinful indulgences. I guarantee that your next glassful will lead to rejoicing, not regretting.

Maintenance Smoothies

———

ULTRA-LOW CARB SMOOTHIES

These smoothies
have *12* grams
of carbohydrates
or less.

Almond Joy Strawberry Smoothie

The Peter Paul Candy Company introduced the ever-popular Almond Joy candy bar in 1948. Today, I hope you'll be equally pleased with the debut of this low-carb smoothie adaptation of their famous sweet. For an extra treat, dip the rim of a cocktail glass in a blend of melted low-carb semisweet chocolate thinned with a dab of canola oil, then place it in the refrigerator or freezer to allow the chocolate to set. Serve this delectable treat in the decked-out glass and wait for the rave reviews.

1 SERVING

¼ cup Carb Countdown (or favorite low-carb)
   dairy beverage
2 tablespoons sugar-free chocolate syrup
2 tablespoons sugar-free coconut syrup
½ cup partially frozen diced strawberries
½ cup low-carb vanilla ice cream

Place all the ingredients in a blender container in the order listed. Place the cover on the container. Turn on the blender and process by pressing the pulse button, while on the lowest blade-speed setting, until the ingredients are mostly blended. Continue mixing without the pulse function by pressing the highest blade-speed

RECIPE CONTINUES

setting button until the mixture is smooth (it may be necessary to turn off the blender periodically and stir the mixture with a spoon, working from the bottom up). Turn off the blender. Pour the smoothie into a glass and garnish with a Chocolate-Dipped Strawberry (page 196), if desired.

Berry Tales

Like the ultra-thin Snow White, Sleeping Beauty, and Cinderella, you can live happily ever after by banishing the evil carb gremlins from your kingdom and enjoying a deliciously slimming smoothie like this one.

1 SERVING

½ cup Old Orchard Lo Carb apple raspberry juice cocktail blend (or favorite low-carb juice)

2 tablespoons sugar-free pineapple syrup

½ cup partially frozen raspberries

¼ cup Blueberry Sorbet (page 179) or favorite low-carb sorbet

½ tablespoon KĒTO (or favorite low-carb) French vanilla instant pudding powder

½ teaspoon sugar-free raspberry Jell-O powder (optional)

Place all the ingredients in a blender container in the order listed. Place the cover on the container. Turn on the blender and process by pressing the pulse button, while on the lowest blade-speed setting, until the ingredients are mostly blended. Continue mixing without the pulse function by pressing the highest blade-speed setting button until the mixture is smooth (it may be necessary to turn off the blender periodically and stir the mixture with a spoon, working from the bottom up). Turn off the blender. Pour the smoothie into a glass and garnish with an Apple Chip (page 187), if desired.

Chocolate Almond Bar Smoothie

In 1908, the Hershey Chocolate Company made the first milk chocolate bar with almonds. Almost a hundred years later, we can now indulge in a low-carb smoothie made with luscious chocolate ice cream, almond flavoring, and sweet strawberries. Wrap the glass in dark brown paper and bring back memories of your high-carb childhood.

1 SERVING

6 tablespoons Carb Countdown
   (or favorite low-carb) dairy beverage
2 tablespoons sugar-free almond syrup
1/2 cup partially frozen diced strawberries
1/2 cup low-carb chocolate ice cream

Place all the ingredients in a blender container in the order listed. Place the cover on the container. Turn on the blender and process by pressing the pulse button, while on the lowest blade-speed setting, until the ingredients are mostly blended. Continue mixing without the pulse function by pressing the highest blade-speed setting button until the mixture is smooth (it may be necessary to turn off the blender periodically and stir the mixture with a spoon, working from the bottom up). Turn off the blender. Pour the smoothie into a glass and garnish with a Chocolate Chip Meringue on a Skewer (page 190), if desired.

Chocolate Blueberry Celebration

Reward yourself with this spectacular low-carb chocolate, strawberry, and blueberry indulgence. For added excitement, serve this delectable treat in a chocolate-rimmed cocktail glass (see Almond Joy Strawberry Smoothie on page 135), but dip the melted chocolate in Splenda before chilling the glass.

1 SERVING

6 tablespoons diet cherry soda
2 tablespoons sugar-free chocolate syrup
1/4 cup partially frozen diced strawberries
1/4 cup partially frozen blueberries
1/2 cup low-carb chocolate ice cream

Place all the ingredients in a blender container in the order listed. Place the cover on the container. Turn on the blender and process by pressing the pulse button, while on the lowest blade-speed setting, until the ingredients are mostly blended. Continue mixing without the pulse function by pressing the highest blade-speed setting button until the mixture is smooth (it may be necessary to turn off the blender periodically and stir the mixture with a spoon, working from the bottom up). Turn off the blender. Pour the smoothie into a glass and garnish with 1 or 2 Chocolate-Dipped Marshmallows (page 194), if desired.

Chocolate Raspberry Extravaganza

This lavish smoothie, made with chocolate, raspberries, ice cream, and pudding, is spectacularly low in carbs but rich in taste.

1 SERVING

1/4 cup strawberry kiwi (or favorite flavor)
  Crystal Light soft drink
2 to 3 tablespoons sugar-free chocolate syrup
2 tablespoons heavy cream
  (or Carb Countdown dairy beverage)
1/2 cup partially frozen raspberries
1/2 cup low-carb vanilla ice cream
1/2 tablespoon KĒTO (or favorite low-carb)
  French vanilla instant pudding powder (optional)

Place all the ingredients in a blender container in the order listed. Place the cover on the container. Turn on the blender and process by pressing the pulse button, while on the lowest blade-speed setting, until the ingredients are mostly blended. Continue mixing without the pulse function by pressing the highest blade-speed setting button until the mixture is smooth (it may be necessary to turn off the blender periodically and stir the mixture with a spoon, working from the bottom up). Turn off the blender. Pour the smoothie into a glass and garnish with a Chocolate Chip Meringue on a Skewer (page 190), if desired.

Chocolate Raspberry Fantasy

Stop dreaming and wake up to the reality of rich chocolate and raspberries in this chilled treat that's guaranteed to satisfy your sweet tooth.

1 SERVING

6 tablespoons chocolate Carb Countdown
   (or favorite low-carb) dairy beverage
2 tablespoons sugar-free almond syrup
½ cup partially frozen raspberries
½ cup low-carb chocolate ice cream

Place all the ingredients in a blender container in the order listed. Place the cover on the container. Turn on the blender and process by pressing the pulse button, while on the lowest blade-speed setting, until the ingredients are mostly blended. Continue mixing without the pulse function by pressing the highest blade-speed setting button until the mixture is smooth (it may be necessary to turn off the blender periodically and stir the mixture with a spoon, working from the bottom up). Turn off the blender. Pour the smoothie into a glass and garnish with a Peanut Butter Cookie on a Skewer (page 201), if desired.

Chocolate Strawberry Madness

Madness, maybe. Badness, no. There are only 10 carbs in this enchanting treat featuring the classic combination of strawberry and chocolate.

1 SERVING

¼ cup strawberry kiwi (or favorite flavor) Crystal Light soft drink

2 tablespoons sugar-free chocolate syrup

2 tablespoons heavy cream (or Carb Countdown dairy beverage)

½ cup partially frozen diced strawberries

½ cup low-carb strawberry ice cream

½ tablespoon KĒTO (or favorite low-carb) French vanilla instant pudding powder (optional)

Place all the ingredients in a blender container in the order listed. Place the cover on the container. Turn on the blender and process by pressing the pulse button, while on the lowest blade-speed setting, until the ingredients are mostly blended. Continue mixing without the pulse function by pressing the highest blade-speed setting button until the mixture is smooth (it may be necessary to turn off the blender periodically and stir the mixture with a spoon, working from the bottom up). Turn off the blender. Pour the smoothie into a glass and garnish with a Chocolate-Dipped Strawberry (page 196), if desired.

Coconut CarbBuster

Who you gonna call when you're hungry for a sweet and satisfying snack with less than 11 carbs? Just dial up this amazing chocolate, coconut, and strawberry creation. You'll be haunted by its taste the rest of the day.

1 SERVING

¼ cup chocolate Carb Countdown
    (or favorite low-carb) dairy beverage
2 tablespoons sugar-free coconut syrup
½ cup partially frozen diced strawberries
½ cup low-carb chocolate ice cream

Place all the ingredients in a blender container in the order listed. Place the cover on the container. Turn on the blender and process by pressing the pulse button, while on the lowest blade-speed setting, until the ingredients are mostly blended. Continue mixing without the pulse function by pressing the highest blade-speed setting button until the mixture is smooth (it may be necessary to turn off the blender periodically and stir the mixture with a spoon, working from the bottom up). Turn off the blender. Pour the smoothie into a glass and serve with a Chocolate-Covered Spoon (page 192), if desired.

A Good Report Carb

If you've done your homework and you know the difference between a regular smoothie and a delicious low-carb smoothie, then you'll agree that this apricot and strawberry creation gets an A+.

1 SERVING

½ cup French vanilla-flavored AdvantEdge
 Carb Control (or favorite low-carb)
 ready-to-drink shake
2 tablespoons sugar-free vanilla syrup
¼ cup partially frozen diced apricot
¼ cup partially frozen diced strawberries
½ cup low-carb vanilla ice cream
½ teaspoon sugar-free strawberry Jell-O powder
 (optional)

Place all the ingredients in a blender container in the order listed. Place the cover on the container. Turn on the blender and process by pressing the pulse button, while on the lowest blade-speed setting, until the ingredients are mostly blended. Continue mixing without the pulse function by pressing the highest blade-speed setting button until the mixture is smooth (it may be necessary to turn off the blender periodically and stir the mixture with a spoon, working from the bottom up). Turn off the blender. Pour the smoothie into a glass and garnish with Berries on a Skewer (page 189), if desired.

Lions, Tigers, and Berries, Oh My!

This strawberry twister will definitely lift you up. Serve it to friends and everyone will agree you're a wizard. It will definitely be the most wicked whip of the feast.

1 SERVING

½ cup creamy vanilla-flavored Atkins Advantage
   (or favorite low-carb) ready-to-drink shake
3 tablespoons sugar-free strawberry syrup
½ cup partially frozen diced strawberries
½ cup low-carb strawberry ice cream

Place all the ingredients in a blender container in the order listed. Place the cover on the container. Turn on the blender and process by pressing the pulse button, while on the lowest blade-speed setting, until the ingredients are mostly blended. Continue mixing without the pulse function by pressing the highest blade-speed setting button until the mixture is smooth (it may be necessary to turn off the blender periodically and stir the mixture with a spoon, working from the bottom up). Turn off the blender. Pour the smoothie into a glass and garnish with a Crisp Strawberry Wafer (page 198), if desired.

Low Dancing

Find a partner to share this tantalizing coconut, strawberry, and chocolate smoothie—or drink it solo.

1 SERVING

6 tablespoons chocolate Carb Countdown
(or favorite low-carb) dairy beverage
2 tablespoons sugar-free coconut syrup
1 tablespoon sugar-free chocolate syrup
½ cup partially frozen diced strawberries
½ cup low-carb vanilla ice cream

Place all the ingredients in a blender container in the order listed. Place the cover on the container. Turn on the blender and process by pressing the pulse button, while on the lowest blade-speed setting, until the ingredients are mostly blended. Continue mixing without the pulse function by pressing the highest blade-speed setting button until the mixture is smooth (it may be necessary to turn off the blender periodically and stir the mixture with a spoon, working from the bottom up). Turn off the blender. Pour the smoothie into a glass and serve with a Chocolate-Covered Spoon (page 192), if desired.

Luxury Carbs

You can enjoy a Mercedes worth of flavor on a Toyota diet with this amazingly plush three-fruit low-carb smoothie featuring strawberry ice cream as standard equipment.

1 SERVING

¼ cup diet cherry soda
2 tablespoons sugar-free blueberry syrup
2 tablespoons heavy cream
 (or Carb Countdown dairy beverage)
¼ cup partially frozen diced strawberries
¼ cup partially frozen blueberries
½ cup low-carb strawberry ice cream
½ teaspoon sugar-free strawberry Jell-O powder
 (optional)

Place all the ingredients in a blender container in the order listed. Place the cover on the container. Turn on the blender and process by pressing the pulse button, while on the lowest blade-speed setting, until the ingredients are mostly blended. Continue mixing without the pulse function by pressing the highest blade-speed setting button until the mixture is smooth (it may be necessary to turn off the blender periodically and stir the mixture with a spoon, working from the bottom up). Turn off the blender. Pour the smoothie into a glass and garnish with a Pecan Cookie on a Skewer (page 203), if desired.

Raspberry Chocolate Espresso

If you're looking for a little magic in your smoothie, you'll be pleased with this coffee-enhanced version.

1 SERVING

6 tablespoons chocolate Carb Countdown
   (or favorite low-carb) dairy beverage
2 tablespoons sugar-free chocolate syrup
1 to 2 tablespoons coffee extract or strong coffee
   (see Note)
½ cup partially frozen raspberries
½ cup low-carb chocolate ice cream

Place all the ingredients in a blender container in the order listed. Place the cover on the container. Turn on the blender and process by pressing the pulse button, while on the lowest blade-speed setting, until the ingredients are mostly blended. Continue mixing without the pulse function by pressing the highest blade-speed setting button until the mixture is smooth (it may be necessary to turn off the blender periodically and stir the mixture with a spoon, working from the bottom up). Turn off the blender. Pour the smoothie into a glass and garnish with a Pecan Cookie on a Skewer (page 203), if desired.

NOTE:
To make strong coffee, dissolve 1 tablespoon of instant coffee powder in 2½ tablespoons of warm water; blend well. Chill for at least 15 minutes.

Razzle-Dazzle Smoothie

You'll be awestruck by how satisfying and delicious a low-carb smoothie can be after tasting this special treat made with raspberries and strawberry ice cream.

1 SERVING

1/4 cup Old Orchard Lo Carb apple raspberry juice cocktail blend (or favorite low-carb juice)

1/2 cup creamy vanilla–flavored Atkins Advantage (or favorite low-carb) ready-to-drink shake

3 tablespoons sugar-free raspberry syrup

1/2 cup partially frozen raspberries

1/2 cup low-carb strawberry ice cream

Place all the ingredients in a blender container in the order listed. Place the cover on the container. Turn on the blender and process by pressing the pulse button, while on the lowest blade-speed setting, until the ingredients are mostly blended. Continue mixing without the pulse function by pressing the highest blade-speed setting button until the mixture is smooth (it may be necessary to turn off the blender periodically and stir the mixture with a spoon, working from the bottom up). Turn off the blender. Pour the smoothie into a glass and garnish with an Apple Chip (page 187), if desired.

Sippin' and Slidin'

You'll surrender after one sip of this delicious raspberry smoothie with blueberry and cherry overtones.

1 SERVING

½ cup diet cherry soda

2 tablespoons sugar-free cherry syrup

2 tablespoons heavy cream (or Carb Countdown dairy beverage)

½ cup partially frozen raspberries

¼ cup partially frozen blueberries

¼ cup Blueberry Sorbet (page 179) or favorite low-carb sorbet

½ tablespoon KĒTO (or favorite low-carb) French vanilla instant pudding powder

½ teaspoon sugar-free cherry Jell-O powder (optional)

Place all the ingredients in a blender container in the order listed. Place the cover on the container. Turn on the blender and process by pressing the pulse button, while on the lowest blade-speed setting, until the ingredients are mostly blended. Continue mixing without the pulse function by pressing the highest blade-speed setting button until the mixture is smooth (it may be necessary to turn off the blender periodically and stir the mixture with a spoon, working from the bottom up). Turn off the blender. Pour the smoothie into a glass and garnish with a Crisp Blueberry Wafer (page 198), if desired.

Slimming with Sharks

There might be a power struggle between you and your mate over who gets the first sip of this strawberry and apricot smoothie. At less than 12 carbs per serving, there's plenty for all, so just dive in and enjoy!

1 SERVING

½ cup creamy vanilla-flavored Atkins Advantage
  (or favorite low-carb) ready-to-drink shake
3 tablespoons sugar-free pineapple syrup
¼ cup partially frozen diced strawberries
3 tablespoons partially frozen diced apricot
½ cup low-carb strawberry ice cream

Place all the ingredients in a blender container in the order listed. Place the cover on the container. Turn on the blender and process by pressing the pulse button, while on the lowest blade-speed setting, until the ingredients are mostly blended. Continue mixing without the pulse function by pressing the highest blade-speed setting button until the mixture is smooth (it may be necessary to turn off the blender periodically and stir the mixture with a spoon, working from the bottom up). Turn off the blender. Pour the smoothie into a glass and garnish the rim with a Strawberry Fan (page 205), if desired.

Strawberry Piña Colada

In the 1950s, a Puerto Rican named Dom Ramón Lopez-Irizarry created coconut cream, made from the tender part of the coconut. A few years later, an inventive bartender experimented by mixing rum and pineapple juice with coconut cream, and the Piña Colada, one of Puerto Rico's favorite drinks, was born. Although this luscious smoothie is made without rum, it still features the same wonderful island flavors.

1 SERVING

$\frac{1}{2}$ cup strawberry kiwi (or favorite flavor) Crystal Light soft drink

2 tablespoons sugar-free pineapple syrup

2 tablespoons sugar-free coconut syrup

$\frac{1}{2}$ cup partially frozen diced strawberries

$\frac{1}{2}$ cup low-carb vanilla ice cream

$\frac{1}{2}$ tablespoon KĒTO (or favorite low-carb) banana instant pudding powder

$\frac{1}{2}$ teaspoon sugar-free strawberry-banana Jell-O powder (optional)

Place all the ingredients in a blender container in the order listed. Place the cover on the container. Turn on the blender and process by pressing the pulse button, while on the lowest blade-speed setting, until the ingredients are mostly blended. Continue mixing without the pulse function by pressing the highest blade-speed setting button until the mixture is smooth (it may be necessary to turn off the blender periodically and stir the mixture with a spoon, working from the bottom up). Turn off the blender. Pour the smoothie into a glass and garnish with a Crisp Strawberry Wafer (page 198), if desired.

Swing Low, Sweet Cherry-ot

If you're sometimes up and sometimes down, this strawberry and kiwi smoothie, laced with cherry flavors, will make every day feel special.

1 SERVING

6 tablespoons diet cherry soda
2 tablespoons sugar-free cherry syrup
2 tablespoons heavy cream
    (or Carb Countdown dairy beverage)
2 tablespoons $\frac{1}{3}$-less-fat cream cheese
$\frac{1}{4}$ cup partially frozen diced kiwi
$\frac{1}{4}$ cup partially frozen diced strawberries
$\frac{1}{4}$ cup Strawberry Sorbet (page 179) or favorite
    low-carb sorbet

Place all the ingredients in a blender container in the order listed. Place the cover on the container. Turn on the blender and process by pressing the pulse button, while on the lowest blade-speed setting, until the ingredients are mostly blended. Continue mixing without the pulse function by pressing the highest blade-speed setting button until the mixture is smooth (it may be necessary to turn off the blender periodically and stir the mixture with a spoon, working from the bottom up). Turn off the blender. Pour the smoothie into a glass and garnish with a Pecan Cookie on a Skewer (page 203), if desired.

Tooth Berry

Don't try putting this delicious raspberry and peach creation under your pillow, but do try enjoying it as a spectacular low-carb snack.

1 SERVING

6 to 8 tablespoons Carb Countdown
   (or favorite low-carb) dairy beverage
3 tablespoons sugar-free coconut syrup
1/4 cup partially frozen raspberries
1/4 cup partially frozen diced peach
1/4 cup Raspberry Sorbet (page 179)
   or favorite low-carb sorbet

Place all the ingredients in a blender container in the order listed. Place the cover on the container. Turn on the blender and process by pressing the pulse button, while on the lowest blade-speed setting, until the ingredients are mostly blended. Continue mixing without the pulse function by pressing the highest blade-speed setting button until the mixture is smooth (it may be necessary to turn off the blender periodically and stir the mixture with a spoon, working from the bottom up). Turn off the blender. Pour the smoothie into a glass and garnish with Berries on a Skewer (page 189), if desired.

Turning Carb-Peels

It's easy to understand why anyone would be excited about indulging in this rich and creamy strawberry and orange smoothie, bursting with flavor.

1 SERVING

¼ cup chocolate Carb Countdown
  (or favorite low-carb) dairy beverage
2 tablespoons sugar-free strawberry syrup
¼ cup partially frozen diced strawberries
¼ cup partially frozen diced orange
½ cup low-carb strawberry ice cream

Place all the ingredients in a blender container in the order listed. Place the cover on the container. Turn on the blender and process by pressing the pulse button, while on the lowest blade-speed setting, until the ingredients are mostly blended. Continue mixing without the pulse function by pressing the highest blade-speed setting button until the mixture is smooth (it may be necessary to turn off the blender periodically and stir the mixture with a spoon, working from the bottom up). Turn off the blender. Pour the smoothie into a glass and garnish with a Chocolate Chip Meringue on a Skewer (page 190), if desired.

Maintenance
Low-Carb Smoothies

———

LOW-CARB SMOOTHIES

These smoothies
have *15* grams
of carbohydrates
or less.

Berry Necessities

You'll need only a few ingredients to whip up this delicious low-carb raspberry and strawberry smoothie.

1 SERVING

1/4 cup Old Orchard Lo Carb apple raspberry juice
    cocktail blend (or favorite low-carb juice)
1/2 cup creamy vanilla-flavored Atkins Advantage
    (or favorite low-carb) ready-to-drink shake
3 tablespoons sugar-free raspberry syrup
1/2 cup partially frozen raspberries
1/2 cup low-carb strawberry ice cream

Place all the ingredients in a blender container in the order listed. Place the cover on the container. Turn on the blender and process by pressing the pulse button, while on the lowest blade-speed setting, until the ingredients are mostly blended. Continue mixing without the pulse function by pressing the highest blade-speed setting button until the mixture is smooth (it may be necessary to turn off the blender periodically and stir the mixture with a spoon, working from the bottom up). Turn off the blender. Pour the smoothie into a glass and garnish with an Apple Chip (page 187), if desired.

Berry Slim Pickins

When the desire to eat something sweet tempts you to "fall off the wagon," hang on, because it takes only minutes to whip up this deliciously satisfying raspberry and blueberry smoothie that will curb the urge and keep you on the low-carb straight and narrow.

1 SERVING

½ cup Minute Maid Light raspberry passion
   (or favorite low-carb) fruit drink
2 tablespoons sugar-free raspberry syrup
2 tablespoons heavy cream
   (or Carb Countdown dairy beverage)
¼ cup partially frozen blueberries
¼ cup partially frozen raspberries
½ tablespoon KĒTO (or favorite low-carb)
   French vanilla instant pudding powder (optional)
½ cup low-carb vanilla ice cream

Place all the ingredients in a blender container in the order listed. Place the cover on the container. Turn on the blender and process by pressing the pulse button, while on the lowest blade-speed setting, until the ingredients are mostly blended. Continue mixing without the pulse function by pressing the highest blade-speed setting button until the mixture is smooth (it may be necessary to turn off the blender periodically and stir the mixture with a spoon, working from the bottom up). Turn off the blender. Pour the smoothie into a glass and garnish with a Crisp Blueberry Wafer (page 198), if desired.

Berry the Hatchet

Let your past mealtime indiscretions be forgotten and just enjoy this wonderful low-carb blueberry and strawberry smoothie.

1 SERVING

½ cup Carb Countdown (or favorite low-carb) dairy beverage

2 tablespoons sugar-free strawberry syrup

½ cup partially frozen diced strawberries

¼ cup partially frozen blueberries

¼ cup Strawberry Sorbet (page 179) or favorite low-carb sorbet

Place all the ingredients in a blender container in the order listed. Place the cover on the container. Turn on the blender and process by pressing the pulse button, while on the lowest blade-speed setting, until the ingredients are mostly blended. Continue mixing without the pulse function by pressing the highest blade-speed setting button until the mixture is smooth (it may be necessary to turn off the blender periodically and stir the mixture with a spoon, working from the bottom up). Turn off the blender. Pour the smoothie into a glass and garnish with Berries on a Skewer (page 189), if desired.

Carb and Driver

This fuel-efficient BMW (Beverage Made Wisely) will provide you with an unbelievable number of smiles per gallon.

1 SERVING

½ cup Carb Countdown (or favorite low-carb) dairy beverage
2 tablespoons sugar-free blueberry syrup
½ cup partially frozen diced strawberries
¼ cup partially frozen blueberries
¼ cup Raspberry Sorbet (page 179) or favorite low-carb sorbet
½ tablespoon KĒTO (or favorite low-carb) French vanilla instant pudding powder

Place all the ingredients in a blender container in the order listed. Place the cover on the container. Turn on the blender and process by pressing the pulse button, while on the lowest blade-speed setting, until the ingredients are mostly blended. Continue mixing without the pulse function by pressing the highest blade-speed setting button until the mixture is smooth (it may be necessary to turn off the blender periodically and stir the mixture with a spoon, working from the bottom up). Turn off the blender. Pour the smoothie into a glass and garnish with a Crisp Strawberry Wafer (page 198), if desired.

Carb-e Diem

Seize the day, not a doughnut. Enjoy satisfying low-carb treats like this tantalizing apple and berry smoothie instead.

1 SERVING

6 tablespoons Old Orchard Lo Carb apple raspberry
  juice cocktail blend (or favorite low-carb juice)
2 tablespoons sugar-free vanilla syrup
6 tablespoons partially frozen raspberries
2 tablespoons partially frozen diced apple
$\frac{1}{2}$ cup low-carb strawberry ice cream

Place all the ingredients in a blender container in the order listed. Place the cover on the container. Turn on the blender and process by pressing the pulse button, while on the lowest blade-speed setting, until the ingredients are mostly blended. Continue mixing without the pulse function by pressing the highest blade-speed setting button until the mixture is smooth (it may be necessary to turn off the blender periodically and stir the mixture with a spoon, working from the bottom up). Turn off the blender. Pour the smoothie into a glass and garnish with an Apple Chip (page 187), if desired.

Chocolate Cable Carbs

If sticking to a bland low-carb diet is too steep a hill to climb, hop aboard, enjoy this peanut butter and chocolate pleaser, and leave your carbs in San Francisco (or Detroit, Peoria, etc.).

1 SERVING

6 tablespoons Carb Countdown
   (or favorite low-carb) dairy beverage
2 tablespoons sugar-free chocolate syrup
1/2 cup partially frozen diced strawberries
1 tablespoon creamy natural peanut butter
1/2 cup low-carb vanilla ice cream

Place all the ingredients in a blender container in the order listed. Place the cover on the container. Turn on the blender and process by pressing the pulse button, while on the lowest blade-speed setting, until the ingredients are mostly blended. Continue mixing without the pulse function by pressing the highest blade-speed setting button until the mixture is smooth (it may be necessary to turn off the blender periodically and stir the mixture with a spoon, working from the bottom up). Turn off the blender. Pour the smoothie into a glass and garnish with a Peanut Butter Cookie on a Skewer (page 201), if desired.

Follow Your Passion Fruit

Now that you're committed to a low-carb diet, go for it with this tropical breeze in a glass. To serve this smoothie with a whimsical touch, first pour some raspberry passion fruit drink in one saucer and Splenda in another. Dip the rim of a cocktail glass in the fruit drink and then the Splenda. Now pour the smoothie into this very chic glass.

1 SERVING

¼ cup Minute Maid Light raspberry passion
   (or favorite low-carb) fruit drink
2 tablespoons sugar-free pineapple syrup
2 tablespoons heavy cream
   (or Carb Countdown dairy beverage)
6 tablespoons partially frozen raspberries
2 tablespoons partially frozen diced banana
¼ cup Raspberry Sorbet (page 179) or favorite
   low-carb sorbet

Place all the ingredients in a blender container in the order listed. Place the cover on the container. Turn on the blender and process by pressing the pulse button, while on the lowest blade-speed setting, until the ingredients are mostly blended. Continue mixing without the pulse function by pressing the highest blade-speed

RECIPE CONTINUES

setting button until the mixture is smooth (it may be necessary to turn off the blender periodically and stir the mixture with a spoon, working from the bottom up). Turn off the blender. Pour the smoothie into a glass and garnish with Berries on a Skewer (page 189), if desired.

Free Chilly

You'll agree that this apricot and blueberry blend is a whale of a refresher. Don't get caught without enough ingredients to net a second serving.

1 SERVING

½ cup Carb Countdown (or favorite low-carb) dairy beverage

2 tablespoons sugar-free mango syrup

¼ cup partially frozen blueberries

¼ cup partially frozen diced apricot

¼ cup Blueberry Sorbet (page 179) or favorite low-carb sorbet

½ tablespoon KĒTO (or favorite low-carb) French vanilla instant pudding powder

Place all the ingredients in a blender container in the order listed. Place the cover on the container. Turn on the blender and process by pressing the pulse button, while on the lowest blade-speed setting, until the ingredients are mostly blended. Continue mixing without the pulse function by pressing the highest blade-speed setting button until the mixture is smooth (it may be necessary to turn off the blender periodically and stir the mixture with a spoon, working from the bottom up). Turn off the blender. Pour the smoothie into a glass and garnish with Berries on a Skewer (page 189), if desired.

Go with the Low

Everyone's doing it. Let yourself be swept along in low-carb ecstasy by sampling this tropical treat featuring mango, strawberry, and apricot.

1 SERVING

6 tablespoons Minute Maid Light mango tropical
     (or favorite low-carb) fruit drink
2 tablespoons sugar-free mango syrup
1/4 cup partially frozen diced strawberries
1/4 cup partially frozen diced apricot
1/2 cup low-carb strawberry ice cream

Place all the ingredients in a blender container in the order listed. Place the cover on the container. Turn on the blender and process by pressing the pulse button, while on the lowest blade-speed setting, until the ingredients are mostly blended. Continue mixing without the pulse function by pressing the highest blade-speed setting button until the mixture is smooth (it may be necessary to turn off the blender periodically and stir the mixture with a spoon, working from the bottom up). Turn off the blender. Pour the smoothie into a glass and garnish with a Peanut Butter Cookie on a Skewer (page 201), if desired.

Gone with the Spin

Carbs, that is. This chocolate and banana masterpiece is a classic that is certain to help your diet and make you a victor in the war between the stouts.

1 SERVING

¼ cup diet cherry soda

2 tablespoons sugar-free chocolate syrup

2 tablespoons heavy cream
   (or Carb Countdown dairy beverage)

¼ cup partially frozen diced strawberries

2 tablespoons partially frozen diced banana

½ cup low-carb vanilla ice cream

Place all the ingredients in a blender container in the order listed. Place the cover on the container. Turn on the blender and process by pressing the pulse button, while on the lowest blade-speed setting, until the ingredients are mostly blended. Continue mixing without the pulse function by pressing the highest blade-speed setting button until the mixture is smooth (it may be necessary to turn off the blender periodically and stir the mixture with a spoon, working from the bottom up). Turn off the blender. Pour the smoothie into a glass and garnish with a Chocolate-Dipped Strawberry (page 196), if desired.

Good-bye, Mr. Hips

It doesn't take a classics scholar to figure out why this flavorful low-carb raspberry and peach smoothie is the perfect way to fight the tape measure.

1 SERVING

6 tablespoons diet cherry soda

2 tablespoons sugar-free banana syrup

2 tablespoons heavy cream
    (or Carb Countdown dairy beverage)

¼ cup partially frozen raspberries

¼ cup partially frozen diced peach

¼ cup Raspberry Sorbet (page 179)
    or favorite low-carb sorbet

½ tablespoon KĒTO (or favorite low-carb)
    French vanilla instant pudding powder

Place all the ingredients in a blender container in the order listed. Place the cover on the container. Turn on the blender and process by pressing the pulse button, while on the lowest blade-speed setting, until the ingredients are mostly blended. Continue mixing without the pulse function by pressing the highest blade-speed setting button until the mixture is smooth (it may be necessary to turn off the blender periodically and stir the mixture with a spoon, working from the bottom up). Turn off the blender. Pour the smoothie into a glass and garnish with Berries on a Skewer (page 189), if desired.

Happily Ever Apple

Blueberries and apples combined in this sensational low-carb smoothie are a marriage made in heaven, a definite cloud nine experience.

1 SERVING

- ¼ cup Old Orchard Lo Carb apple raspberry juice cocktail blend (or favorite low-carb juice)
- 2 tablespoons sugar-free blueberry syrup
- 2 tablespoons heavy cream (or Carb Countdown dairy beverage)
- 6 tablespoons partially frozen blueberries
- 2 tablespoons partially frozen diced apple
- ¼ cup Strawberry Sorbet (page 179) or favorite low-carb sorbet
- ½ teaspoon sugar-free raspberry Jell-O powder (optional)

Place all the ingredients in a blender container in the order listed. Place the cover on the container. Turn on the blender and process by pressing the pulse button, while on the lowest blade-speed setting, until the ingredients are mostly blended. Continue mixing without the pulse function by pressing the highest blade-speed setting button until the mixture is smooth (it may be necessary to turn off the blender periodically and stir the mixture with a spoon, working from the bottom up). Turn off the blender. Pour the smoothie into a glass and garnish with an Apple Chip (page 187), if desired.

Just Say Low!

Don't let friends tempt you with a high-carb trip. Tell 'em Nancy told you to just say no, and stay true to your low-carb lifestyle with this kiwi and passion fruit upper.

1 SERVING

6 tablespoons Minute Maid Light raspberry passion (or favorite low-carb) fruit drink
2 tablespoons sugar-free raspberry syrup
2 tablespoons heavy cream (or Carb Countdown dairy beverage)
¼ cup partially frozen diced kiwi
¼ cup partially frozen blueberries
¼ cup Strawberry Sorbet (page 179) or favorite low-carb sorbet

Place all the ingredients in a blender container in the order listed. Place the cover on the container. Turn on the blender and process by pressing the pulse button, while on the lowest blade-speed setting, until the ingredients are mostly blended. Continue mixing without the pulse function by pressing the highest blade-speed setting button until the mixture is smooth (it may be necessary to turn off the blender periodically and stir the mixture with a spoon, working from the bottom up). Turn off the blender. Pour the smoothie into a glass and garnish with a Crisp Blueberry Wafer (page 198), if desired.

Kiwi Pudding on the Ritz

The Ritz? Not crackers or Carlton, but a great smoothie featuring bananas, strawberries, and kiwi with a touch of pudding.

1 SERVING

6 tablespoons Old Orchard Lo Carb apple raspberry
    juice cocktail blend (or favorite low-carb juice)
2 tablespoons sugar-free banana syrup
1/4 cup partially frozen diced strawberries
1/4 cup partially frozen diced kiwi
1/2 tablespoon KĒTO (or favorite low-carb)
    banana instant pudding powder
1/2 cup low-carb strawberry ice cream

Place all the ingredients in a blender container in the order listed. Place the cover on the container. Turn on the blender and process by pressing the pulse button, while on the lowest blade-speed setting, until the ingredients are mostly blended. Continue mixing without the pulse function by pressing the highest blade-speed setting button until the mixture is smooth (it may be necessary to turn off the blender periodically and stir the mixture with a spoon, working from the bottom up). Turn off the blender. Pour the smoothie into a glass and garnish with an Apple Chip (page 187), if desired.

Low and Behold!
A Strawberry Smoothie

Who would believe that a low-carb dieter could indulge in a smoothie as rich as this ice cream–based creation made with strawberries and banana!

1 SERVING

¼ cup strawberry kiwi (or favorite flavor) Crystal Light soft drink
2 tablespoons sugar-free banana or strawberry syrup
6 tablespoons partially frozen diced strawberries
2 tablespoons partially frozen diced banana
½ cup low-carb strawberry ice cream

Place all the ingredients in a blender container in the order listed. Place the cover on the container. Turn on the blender and process by pressing the pulse button, while on the lowest blade-speed setting, until the ingredients are mostly blended. Continue mixing without the pulse function by pressing the highest blade-speed setting button until the mixture is smooth (it may be necessary to turn off the blender periodically and stir the mixture with a spoon, working from the bottom up). Turn off the blender. Pour the smoothie into a glass and garnish with a Pecan Cookie on a Skewer (page 203), if desired.

Low, Low, Low Your Float

Merrily, merrily, merrily, merrily lite is not a dream.

1 SERVING

¼ cup strawberry kiwi (or favorite flavor) Crystal Light soft drink

2 to 3 tablespoons sugar-free peach syrup

½ cup low-carb peach yogurt

¼ cup partially frozen diced nectarine

¼ cup partially frozen diced kiwi

½ tablespoon KĒTO (or favorite low-carb) French vanilla instant pudding powder

½ teaspoon sugar-free peach Jell-O powder (optional)

Place all the ingredients in a blender container in the order listed. Place the cover on the container. Turn on the blender and process by pressing the pulse button, while on the lowest blade-speed setting, until the ingredients are mostly blended. Continue mixing without the pulse function by pressing the highest blade-speed setting button until the mixture is smooth (it may be necessary to turn off the blender periodically and stir the mixture with a spoon, working from the bottom up). Turn off the blender. Pour the smoothie into a glass and garnish with a Pear Chip (page 187), if desired.

Peanut Butter Cup Smoothie

In the 1920s, the H. B. Reese Candy Company introduced peanut butter cups made with specially processed peanut butter and Hershey's milk chocolate, known today as Reese's Peanut Butter Cups. Try this low-carb smoothie version of the popular candy treat, featuring the added flavor of raspberries.

1 SERVING

6 tablespoons Carb Countdown
　(or favorite low-carb) dairy beverage
2 tablespoons sugar-free almond syrup
½ cup partially frozen raspberries
1 tablespoon creamy natural peanut butter
½ cup low-carb chocolate ice cream

Place all the ingredients in a blender container in the order listed. Place the cover on the container. Turn on the blender and process by pressing the pulse button, while on the lowest blade-speed setting, until the ingredients are mostly blended. Continue mixing without the pulse function by pressing the highest blade-speed setting button until the mixture is smooth (it may be necessary to turn off the blender periodically and stir the mixture with a spoon, working from the bottom up). Turn off the blender. Pour the smoothie into a glass and garnish with a Peanut Butter Cookie on a Skewer (page 201), if desired.

The Pride and the Passion Fruit

You won't be ashamed to serve this amazing smoothie featuring passion fruit combined with the flavors of three other fruits.

1 SERVING

$\frac{1}{2}$ cup Minute Maid Light raspberry passion
  (or favorite low-carb) fruit drink
3 tablespoons sugar-free blueberry syrup
$\frac{1}{4}$ cup partially frozen diced strawberries
$\frac{1}{4}$ cup partially frozen blueberries
2 tablespoons partially frozen diced banana
$\frac{1}{2}$ cup low-carb vanilla ice cream

Place all the ingredients in a blender container in the order listed. Place the cover on the container. Turn on the blender and process by pressing the pulse button, while on the lowest blade-speed setting, until the ingredients are mostly blended. Continue mixing without the pulse function by pressing the highest blade-speed setting button until the mixture is smooth (it may be necessary to turn off the blender periodically and stir the mixture with a spoon, working from the bottom up). Turn off the blender. Pour the smoothie into a glass and garnish with a Crisp Blueberry Wafer (page 198), if desired.

Strawberry Blueberry Bling Bling

Go ahead and show off this glistening gem of a low-carb smoothie.

1 SERVING

¼ cup strawberry kiwi (or favorite flavor)
    Crystal Light soft drink
3 tablespoons sugar-free blueberry syrup
½ cup creamy vanilla–flavored Atkins Advantage
    (or favorite low-carb) ready-to-drink shake
¼ cup partially frozen blueberries
¼ cup partially frozen raspberries
½ cup low-carb strawberry ice cream

Place all the ingredients in a blender container in the order listed. Place the cover on the container. Turn on the blender and process by pressing the pulse button, while on the lowest blade-speed setting, until the ingredients are mostly blended. Continue mixing without the pulse function by pressing the highest blade-speed setting button until the mixture is smooth (it may be necessary to turn off the blender periodically and stir the mixture with a spoon, working from the bottom up). Turn off the blender. Pour the smoothie into a glass and garnish with a Crisp Strawberry Wafer (page 198), if desired.

Strawberry, Raspberry, or Blueberry Sorbet

This recipe for sorbet is adapted from my cookbook *101 Great Lowfat Desserts*. This icy delight adds both flavor and consistency when included in many of the low-carb smoothies found throughout this book. Enjoy!

1½ CUPS SORBET

BASIC SYRUP
1 cup Splenda
1 cup cold water

SORBET
2 cups strawberries (hulled and quartered), raspberries, or blueberries
⅓ cup Basic Syrup
¼ teaspoon fresh lemon juice

To make the **Basic Syrup,** combine the Splenda and water in a heavy, medium saucepan over moderate heat and bring to a boil, stirring occasionally; simmer for 1 minute. Remove the saucepan from the heat. Allow the syrup to cool to room temperature before storing it in a covered container in the refrigerator. The syrup should be very cold before you add it to the strawberries.

To make the **Sorbet,** place the strawberries (raspberries, or blueberries) in the workbowl of a food processor fitted with a metal blade and purée. Add the Basic Syrup and lemon juice and blend well.

RECIPE CONTINUES

Transfer the mixture to an ice cube tray and freeze for 2 hours, or until almost firm (you should be able to easily pierce a fruit cube with the point of a knife). Transfer the fruit cubes to the workbowl of a food processor fitted with a metal blade and process until smooth. Spoon the sorbet into a covered container and freeze until needed.

If the sorbet is too firm when you are ready to use it, allow it to sit at room temperature for 15 to 20 minutes. Alternatively, the sorbet can be warmed in a microwave on High for 30 seconds.

Uptown Whirl

This classy strawberry and blueberry smoothie is rich in flavor yet surprising low in carbs.

1 SERVING

6 tablespoons Carb Countdown
    (or favorite low-carb) dairy beverage
2 tablespoons sugar-free blueberry syrup
¼ cup partially frozen diced strawberries
2 tablespoons partially frozen blueberries
1 tablespoon creamy natural peanut butter
½ cup low-carb strawberry ice cream

Place all the ingredients in a blender container in the order listed. Place the cover on the container. Turn on the blender and process by pressing the pulse button, while on the lowest blade-speed setting, until the ingredients are mostly blended. Continue mixing without the pulse function by pressing the highest blade-speed setting button until the mixture is smooth (it may be necessary to turn off the blender periodically and stir the mixture with a spoon, working from the bottom up). Turn off the blender. Pour the smoothie into a glass and garnish with a Peanut Butter Cookie on a Skewer (page 201), if desired.

The Whirl from Ipanema

This strawberry and blueberry smoothie is a Rio taste treat.

1 SERVING

1/4 cup Old Orchard Lo Carb apple raspberry juice
    cocktail blend (or favorite low-carb juice)
2 tablespoons sugar-free vanilla syrup
2 tablespoons heavy cream
    (or Carb Countdown dairy beverage)
1/2 cup partially frozen diced strawberries
1/4 cup partially frozen blueberries
1/2 cup low-carb strawberry ice cream

Place all the ingredients in a blender container in the order listed. Place the cover on the container. Turn on the blender and process by pressing the pulse button, while on the lowest blade-speed setting, until the ingredients are mostly blended. Continue mixing without the pulse function by pressing the highest blade-speed setting button until the mixture is smooth (it may be necessary to turn off the blender periodically and stir the mixture with a spoon, working from the bottom up). Turn off the blender. Pour the smoothie into a glass and garnish the rim with a Strawberry Fan (page 205), if desired.

You Blue It!

Had a double cheeseburger with fries yesterday? Not to worry. You can make amends today with this delectable and guilt-free blueberry, kiwi, and banana creation.

1 SERVING

6 tablespoons diet cherry soda
2 tablespoons sugar-free banana syrup
2 tablespoons heavy cream
    (or Carb Countdown dairy beverage)
$\frac{1}{4}$ cup partially frozen diced kiwi
$\frac{1}{4}$ cup partially frozen blueberries
$\frac{1}{4}$ cup Blueberry Sorbet (page 179)
    or favorite low-carb sorbet
$\frac{1}{2}$ teaspoon sugar-free cherry Jell-O powder
    (optional)

Place all the ingredients in a blender container in the order listed. Place the cover on the container. Turn on the blender and process by pressing the pulse button, while on the lowest blade-speed setting, until the ingredients are mostly blended. Continue mixing without the pulse function by pressing the highest blade-speed setting button until the mixture is smooth (it may be necessary to turn off the blender periodically and stir the mixture with a spoon, working from the bottom up). Turn off the blender. Pour the smoothie into a glass and garnish with a Crisp Blueberry Wafer (page 198), if desired.

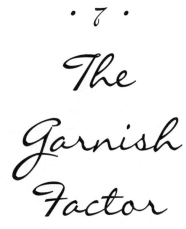

• 7 •

The Garnish Factor

How to Embellish a Low-Carb Smoothie

Garnishes must be matched like a tie to a suit.

—FERNAND POINT (1897–1955)
Ma Gastronomie

SMOOTHIES ARE MORE KNOWN FOR THEIR unique combinations of flavors and textures than for their appearance, but when the occasion calls for it, a well-chosen garnish can create something striking out of an otherwise simple combination of ingredients. Whether you choose a basic garnish, such as a Strawberry Fan, or a more elaborate embellishment, such as a Pecan Cookie on a Skewer, to adorn your smoothie, the added colors and shapes can result in a creation that will impress your family and guests. What's more, most of these garnishes are themselves exceptionally delicious, and all are low-carb.

In this chapter, you will find a host of novel ideas for garnishes that will add a whimsical touch to your low-carb smoothies. Most are not very complicated to make. You can choose to make many garnishes well in advance, and some can even be kept frozen so you'll have a ready supply available for an instant smoothie celebration. On the other hand, if you don't have the time or inclination to make your own garnishes, consider picking up some fun accessories at your neighborhood party store, such as multicolored and uniquely shaped straws, cocktail umbrellas, brightly colored metallic sparklers, paper flowers, or fancy swizzle sticks.

When you are following a low-carb diet plan, garnishing a smoothie may seem to be the last thing you want to think (or care) about. I am convinced that once you've served one artfully decorated with a colorful and tasty embellishment, you'll become a convert. This added touch of whimsy will not only impress, it will reinforce the notion that following a low-carb diet can be fun, rewarding, and deliciously exciting.

Apple or Pear Chips

These chips are crunchy, paper-thin slices of apples or pears. They are the perfect garnish to dress up any smoothie. Not only do they add a sophisticated elegance to smoothies, they are delicious as well. The chips are best when the apples or pears are thinly sliced with a mandoline or vegetable slicer; however, with a little patience, a sharp knife can be almost as effective.

16 TO 20 CHIPS

1 Granny Smith or Golden Delicious apple
   (or firm pear), unpeeled and uncored
4 cups cold water
¼ cup fresh lemon juice
2 cups Splenda

Preheat the oven to 200°F. Line a baking sheet with a silicone baking mat.

Thinly slice the apple into horizontal slices, about ¹⁄₁₆ inch thick, or as thin as possible (remove and discard any seeds). Place the apple slices in a bowl with 2 cups of the water and 2 tablespoons of the lemon juice. Set aside.

Bring the Splenda and the remaining 2 cups of water and 2 tablespoons of lemon juice to a boil in a large saucepan over medium-high heat, stirring fre-

RECIPE CONTINUES

quently to dissolve the Splenda. Using tongs, transfer the apple slices, one slice at a time, to the saucepan and cook for 1 to 2 minutes, or until the mixture returns to a boil.

Using tongs, remove the apple slices from the syrup and place them in a single layer on the prepared baking sheet. Pat both sides of the slices dry with a double layer of paper towels. Bake the apple slices for 1 hour, or until they are dry and crisp. (To test for doneness, remove an apple slice from the baking sheet and allow it to cool. If it is not crisp, bake the slices a little longer, checking every 15 minutes to see if they're done.) Remove the apple chips from the pan and place them on a wire rack to cool completely. The finished chips can be stored in an airtight container in a cool, dry place for up to 2 weeks.

Berries on a Skewer

This beautiful, yet easy-to-prepare garnish adds a rich color that complements most smoothies.

2 SKEWERS OF BERRIES

½ cup fresh raspberries, blueberries, or blackberries
2 6- to 10-inch wooden skewers

Thread 5 to 6 berries of your choice onto the upper half of each skewer. The berries on a skewer can be stored in an airtight container (or placed on a plate and covered with plastic wrap) in the refrigerator for up to 2 days.

Chocolate Chip Meringue on a Skewer

These sweet gems are delicious low-carb treats that add both flavor and flair to a low-carb smoothie. The cookies can also be made into a sandwichlike treat by spreading melted low-carb semisweet or milk chocolate (see Chocolate-Dipped Strawberry on page 196) on the bottom of one cookie and topping it with the bottom of another.

12 TO 16 SKEWERS OF MERINGUES

2 large egg whites, at room temperature
½ cup Splenda
⅛ teaspoon coarse salt (optional)
½ teaspoon pure vanilla extract
½ cup zero-carb (or low-carb) semisweet or milk chocolate chips
12 to 16 10-inch wooden skewers

Preheat the oven to 350°F. Line a baking sheet with parchment paper. Set aside.

Place the egg whites in the mixing bowl of an electric mixer and beat on medium-high speed until foamy. Gradually add the Splenda, and salt, if using, and beat on medium-high speed until stiff; then add the vanilla, ¼ teaspoon at a time, and blend well. Increase the speed to high and beat for 3 to 4 minutes, or until very stiff. Fold in the chocolate chips. Use a 2-tablespoon ice cream scoop or large spoon to drop the meringues onto the prepared baking sheet, spaced 2 inches apart. Place the baking sheet in the oven and bake for 45 minutes, or until the meringues lift off the paper. Remove the cookie sheet from the oven and place it on a cooling rack. Allow the meringues to cool completely before storing them in an airtight container at room temperature for up to 2 weeks. When ready to serve, insert a wooden skewer halfway into the center of each cookie and place it upright in the smoothie.

Chocolate-Covered Spoon

These whimsical chocolate-covered spoons add a delicious touch when serving a low-carb smoothie.

3 TO 4 SPOONS

1/4 cup zero-carb (or low-carb) semisweet or
   milk chocolate chips
1/4 to 1/2 teaspoon (or more) canola oil
3 to 4 plastic teaspoons
4 feet gold cord for bow (optional)

Line a baking sheet with wax paper. Set aside.

Place the chocolate chips in a small saucepan, covered, over very low heat. Cook, stirring occasionally, until the chocolate has melted. (The chocolate can also be placed in a small dish or 5-ounce ramekin, covered with plastic wrap, and set on the hot plate of a coffeemaker. Turn on the coffeemaker, and the chocolate will slowly melt. Stir occasionally.) Remove the chocolate from the heat and whisk in the canola oil, 1/4 teaspoon at a time, until the chocolate is smooth and thin enough to coat the spoons.

Dip the bowl of each spoon in melted chocolate and shake gently to remove any excess. Place the spoons on the prepared baking sheet (or upright in a short glass). Allow the spoons to sit at room temperature for 2 to 3 hours to let the chocolate harden, then tie the optional gold cord into a bow around the upper part of each handle just below the bowl of the spoon. If the chocolate-dipped spoons are not going to be served right away, they can be stored in an airtight container at room temperature for up to 2 days.

Chocolate-Dipped Marshmallow

These chocolate-dipped marshmallows are fabulous as a garnish when one or two are inserted upright into a smoothie.

8 MARSHMALLOWS

$\frac{1}{4}$ cup zero-carb (or low-carb) semisweet or
   milk chocolate chips
$\frac{1}{4}$ to $\frac{1}{2}$ teaspoon (or more) canola oil
8 low-carb marshmallows
8 6- to 10-inch skewers

Place the chocolate chips in a small saucepan, covered, over very low heat. Cook, stirring occasionally, until the chocolate has melted. (The chocolate can also be placed in a small dish or 5-ounce ramekin, covered with plastic wrap, and set on the hot plate of a coffeemaker. Turn on the coffeemaker and the chocolate will slowly melt. Stir occasionally.) Remove the chocolate from the heat and whisk in the canola oil, $\frac{1}{4}$ teaspoon at a time, until the chocolate is smooth and thin enough to coat the marshmallows.

Place a marshmallow on a skewer so it is firmly in place without the point sticking through the top. Holding onto the free end of the skewer, dip the top half of the marshmallow into the chocolate, allowing the excess to drip back into the pan while gently twisting the skewer with the marshmallow in the upside-down position. Next, turn the skewer so the marshmallow is pointing up and place the free end of the skewer into a glass so the marshmallow can dry without touching anything. Repeat with the remaining marshmallows. Allow the marshmallows to sit at room temperature for 2 to 3 hours to let the chocolate harden. If the chocolate-dipped marshmallows are not going to be served right away, remove the skewers. Store the marshmallows in an airtight container at room temperature for up to 1 week. When ready to serve, insert a skewer into the marshmallow and place it upright in a smoothie. (The marshmallows can also be refrigerated immediately after dipping to let the chocolate harden. These marshmallows should be stored in an airtight container in the refrigerator.)

Chocolate-Dipped Strawberry

These strawberries are a delicious way to dress up any smoothie. They also make a fabulous low-carb snack when eaten alone.

2 TO 4 STRAWBERRIES

¼ cup zero-carb (or low-carb) semisweet or
   milk chocolate chips
¼ to ½ teaspoon (or more) canola oil
2 to 4 strawberries
2 6- to 10-inch wooden skewers

Line a baking sheet with wax paper. Set aside.

Wash the berries, then pat them dry with a paper towel. Place them on a dry paper towel and let them sit at room temperature until needed.

Place the chocolate chips in a small saucepan, covered, over very low heat. Cook, stirring occasionally, until the chocolate has melted. (The chocolate can also be placed in a small dish or 5-ounce ramekin, covered with plastic wrap, and set on the hot plate of a coffeemaker. Turn on the coffeemaker and the chocolate will slowly melt. Stir occasionally.) Remove the chocolate from the heat and whisk in the canola oil, ¼ teaspoon at a time, until the chocolate is smooth and thin enough to coat the strawberries.

Make sure the strawberries are completely dry and at room temperature before dipping. Dip the pointed end of each strawberry into the chocolate, halfway up, allowing the excess to drip back into the pan. Place the dipped strawberries on the prepared baking sheet and refrigerate for 5 to 10 minutes to let the chocolate harden. The strawberries can be stored at room temperature for up to 24 hours. When ready to serve, insert a wooden skewer halfway into the center of each strawberry and place it upright in the smoothie.

Crisp Blueberry or Strawberry Wafer

These crispy wafers are simply made of puréed blueberries or strawberries blended with Splenda for added sweetness. They are baked in a slow oven until the mixture becomes crisp. When cool, they are broken into irregular pieces that can be used to adorn any of the smoothies found in this book.

16 TO 20 CRISP WAFERS

1 cup blueberries (or halved and hulled strawberries)
1 tablespoon Splenda

Preheat the oven to 200°F. Line a baking sheet with a silicone baking mat.

Place the blueberries and Splenda in the workbowl of a food processor fitted with a metal blade (or in a blender) and process for 45 seconds, or until the fruit is puréed. Spoon the puréed blueberries in the center of the prepared baking sheet. Using an angular metal spatula (or straight spatula), spread the purée evenly over the mat into a rectangular shape, about $1/16$ inch thick, making sure the purée is thin but not transparent. Place the baking sheet in the oven and bake the blueberry purée for $2\frac{1}{2}$ to 3 hours, or until completely dry and crisp. Remove the pan from the oven, place another baking sheet over the baked blueberries, and invert the pan. Gently remove the silicone baking mat and allow the baked blueberries to cool for 30 minutes to an hour. When the baked blueberries are cool, break them into irregular triangular shapes. The crisp blueberry wafers can be stored in an airtight container at room temperature for up to 2 weeks.

Orange or Lime Wheel

If you are fortunate enough to have a garnishing set that includes a food decorator tool or canalling knife, follow the instrument's instructions. If these tools are unavailable or you are simply possessed of the pioneer spirit, then you will find that the technique for making fruit wheels described below, taught to me by my mother, is quite simple and requires only a fork.

5 TO 6 WHEELS

1 orange or lime

Using a fork, start at one end of the fruit and move the fork down to the other end, slightly piercing the peel. Repeat this process around the entire fruit. Remove the ends and cut the fruit into ¼-inch-thick vertical slices. Store the orange or lime wheels in an airtight container in the refrigerator for up to 2 days. To hang the wheel over the rim of a glass, make a slit by cutting through the peel and halfway into the flesh. Fit the slit over the rim of the glass.

Peanut Butter Cookie on a Skewer

If you love peanut butter, then these peanutty cookies, with only three simple ingredients, are a quick and tasty way to satisfy your craving for something chewy to complement your low-carb smoothie.

20 TO 22 COOKIES

1 cup creamy natural peanut butter
1 cup Splenda
1 large egg
20 to 22 10-inch wooden skewers

Preheat the oven to 325°F. Line a baking sheet with parchment paper.

Using a handheld mixer (or an upright mixer), beat the peanut butter, Splenda, and egg in a medium bowl until well blended, scraping down the sides of the bowl with a rubber spatula as necessary. Pinch off a heaping tablespoon of the peanut butter mixture and roll it between the palms of your hands to form a round ball. Repeat this process with the remaining mixture and place each ball on the prepared baking sheet, spaced 2 inches apart. Place the baking sheet in the oven and bake for 8 to 10 minutes, or until the peanut butter cookies are slightly firm to the touch. Remove the baking sheet from the oven and place it on a cooling rack. Cool completely. Store the peanut

RECIPE CONTINUES

butter cookies in an airtight container in the refrigerator or at room temperature for up to 2 weeks. When ready to serve, insert a wooden skewer halfway into the center of each cookie and place it upright in a smoothie.

Pecan Cookie on a Skewer

These low-carb pecan cookies are decadently sweet and almost melt in your mouth. They make a sensationally delicious garnish when a skewer is inserted into each one and placed upright in a smoothie. One more trick is to dip one half of the cooled cookie in melted low-carb semisweet or milk chocolate (see Chocolate-Dipped Strawberry on page 196). How's that for low-carb decadence?

16 TO 18 COOKIES

1 cup high gluten flour
²/₃ cup vanilla whey protein powder
²/₃ cup finely chopped pecans
¹/₈ teaspoon coarse salt
1 cup (2 sticks) unsalted butter, at room temperature
¹/₃ cup Splenda
1 teaspoon pure vanilla extract
16 to 18 10-inch wooden skewers

Preheat the oven to 350°F. Line a baking sheet with parchment paper. Set aside.

Combine the gluten flour, protein powder, pecans, and salt in a medium bowl and blend with a wire whisk.

Place the butter and Splenda in the mixing bowl of an electric mixer (or a handheld mixer) and beat

RECIPE CONTINUES

on medium-high speed for 3 minutes, scraping down the sides of the bowl with a rubber spatula as necessary. Add the vanilla and blend. On medium-low speed, add the dry ingredients and mix until the dough begins to stick together (it will not be a smooth dough). Using your hands, work the dough just until it holds together. Pinch off a heaping tablespoon of the cookie mixture and roll it between the palms of your hands to form a round ball. Repeat this process with the remaining mixture and place each ball on the prepared baking sheet, spaced 2 inches apart. Place the baking sheet in the oven and bake for 14 to 15 minutes, or just until the edges of the pecan cookies begin to brown. Remove the baking sheet from the oven and place it on a cooling rack. Cool completely. Store the pecan cookies in an airtight container at room temperature or in the refrigerator for up to 2 weeks (or they can be frozen for up to 2 months). When ready to serve, insert a wooden skewer halfway into the center of each cookie and place it upright in a smoothie.

Strawberry Fan

Strawberry fans add a nice touch of color when placed on the rim of a glass and are a tasty treat as well.

2 FANS

2 whole firm strawberries, unhulled

Using a very sharp knife, make about 5 to 6 very thin vertical cuts through the strawberry, starting ¼ inch down from the stem end and cutting through to the pointed end. Place the strawberry on a plate and carefully spread the slices apart to resemble an opened fan. Store the strawberry fans in an airtight container in the refrigerator for up to 1 day. When ready to serve, slip a strawberry fan over the rim of each glass.

Mail-Order and Online Shopping

Where to Get Low-Carb Ingredients

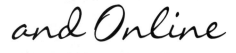

MOST OF THE SUGGESTED LOW-CARB PRODUCTS found in the recipes throughout this book are available in the health section of major supermarkets, as well as in health-food stores and pharmacies. If you cannot find any of these items, there are several online low-carb stores, and most of them also provide a phone or fax number. Here are just a few of these sources.

ALACARB
alacarb.com
orders@alacarb.com
Atkins and KĒTO products, chocolate, and marshmallows

ALLSTARHEALTH
allstarhealth.com
800-875-0448
AdvantEdge Carb Control shakes can also be
purchased in the health section of most supermarkets.
AdvantEdge Carb Control shakes

NDS (NUTRITIONAL DELIVERY SYSTEM)
www.releaseprogram.com
866-820-5559, ext. 115 (ask for Rebecca)
Release can also be purchased at some
GNC stores.
Amplify by Release dietary supplement

DA VINCI
davincigourmet.com
Da Vinci Gourmet, Ltd.
7224 First Avenue South
Seattle, WA 98108
206-768-7401 • 800-640-6779
(Fax) 206-764-3989
Sugar-free syrups

DIET MART
dietmart.com
Atkins and Zone products

DRUGSTORE.COM
drugstore.com
800-DRUGSTORE (800-378-4786)
Atkins and Zone products

LOW CARB

lowcarb.com
lowcarb@dietformulas.com
Atkins products

LOWCARBCUTTERS

lowcarbcutters.com
Customer Service Department
104 Thompson Boulevard
Coldwater, MI 49036
517-677-9520
customerservice@lowcarbcutters.com
Sugar-free syrups and Atkins and KĒTO products

LOW CARB NEXUS

lowcarbnexus.com
A Division of Bailey Ventures, Inc.
3208 East Kivett Drive
High Point, NC 27260
336-887-8606   •   866-526-3987
(Fax) 336-887-8610
Sugar-free syrups, chocolate bars, Atkins and KĒTO products, and whey protein

LOW CARB OUTFITTERS

lowcarboutfitters.com
customerservice@lowcarboutfitters.com
Sugar-free syrups, Atkins and KĒTO products, whey protein, and chocolate chips

LOW CARB OUTLET.COM

lowcarboutlet.com
866-9NO-CARB (866-966-2272)
9:30 A.M.–4:30 P.M. M–F EST

LowCarbOutlet@aol.com
Sugar-free syrups and Atkins and KĒTO products

MONIN
moninstore.com
Sugar-free syrups

NETRITION
netrition.com
888-817-2411   •   (Fax) 518-456-9673
*Chocolate chips, sugar-free syrups, and KĒTO,
Atkins, and Zone products*

TORANI
torani.com
800-775-1925   •   650-875-1200
(Fax) 650-875-1600
Sugar-free syrups

THE VITAMIN BIN
thevitaminbin.com
800-817-7724
Atkins and Zone products

Index

INTERNATIONAL CONVERSION CHART

These are not exact equivalents; they have been slightly rounded to make measuring easier.

Liquid Measurements

AMERICAN	IMPERIAL	METRIC	AUSTRALIAN
2 tbs (1 oz.)	1 fl oz.	30 ml	1 tb
¼ cup (2 oz.)	2 fl. oz.	60 ml	2 tbs
⅓ cup (3 oz.)	3 fl. oz.	80 ml	¼ cup
½ cup (4 oz.)	4 fl. oz.	125 ml	⅓ cup
⅔ cup (5 oz.)	5 fl. oz.	165 ml	½ cup
¾ cup (6 oz.)	6 fl. oz.	185 ml	⅔ cup
1 cup (8 oz.)	8 fl. oz.	250 ml	¾ cup

Spoon Measurements

AMERICAN	METRIC
¼ teaspoon	1 ml
½ teaspoon	2 ml
1 teaspoon	5 ml
1 tablespoon	15 ml

Weights

US/UK	METRIC	US/UK	METRIC
1 oz.	30 grams (g)	8 oz. (½ lb)	250 g
2 oz.	60 g	10 oz.	315 g
4 oz. (¼ lb)	125 g	12 oz.	375 g
5 oz. (⅓ lb)	155 g	14 oz.	440 g
6 oz.	185 g	16 oz. (1 lb)	500 g
7 oz.	220 g	2 lbs	1 kg

Oven Temperatures

FAHRENHEIT	CENTIGRADE	GAS
250	120	½
300	150	2
325	160	3
350	180	4
375	190	5
400	200	6
450	230	8

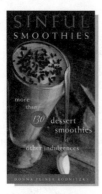
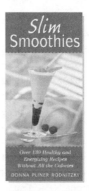
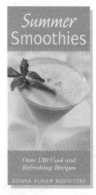
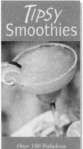
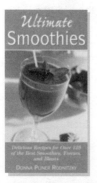